a patient guide

Less Pain and Faster Recovery

Robotic Hysterectomy

The da Vinci® Robotic Surgical System

By

Lennox Hoyte, MD
Abraham Shashoua, MD

Published by MWP Media
30092 Alicia Parkway, Laguna Niguel, CA 92677

Cover designed by Rod Laverne

ISBN 0982878273
Printed in the United States of America

Acknowledgements

The authors wish to thank all those who helped to prepare this book for patient awareness of the latest and least invasive Hysterectomy surgery.

Ms. Grace Hoyte for photo of the first author; Intuitive Surgical (manufactures of the da Vinci Robotic System), for permission to us selected images of the robotic system; Sally Johnson editor.

Table of Contents

Part 1

Hysterectomy and the *da Vinci*® Robotic Surgery System

1

HYSTERECTOMY

One in three women in the U.S. will have a hysterectomy, or surgical removal of the uterus, before the age of 60. The uterus is the hollow, muscular organ that holds and feeds a fertilized egg. Hysterectomy may be done to treat the following conditions that affect the uterus:

- Uterine fibroids
- Endometriosis
- Pelvic support problems (such as uterine prolapse, cystocele, rectocele, and enterocele)
- Abnormal uterine bleeding
- Cancer
- Chronic pelvic pain

When a woman has a medical condition that affects her uterus, the emotional impact can often be as challenging as the physical. Hysterectomy is major surgery and carries some risks. For some conditions, other treatment options are available. However, hysterectomy may offer the best solution. While no woman wants to face surgery, medical technology has dramatically changed the surgical landscape, especially in gynecology. When surgery is needed, the new *da Vinci®* Robotic system is the least traumatic surgical alternative, and may be the most effective treatment for a range of gynecologic problems.

Surgeries that were once performed through large incisions are now being performed with a minimally invasive approach, which benefits patients through a dramatic reduction in trauma, post-operative pain, and recovery time. The vast majority of gynecologic conditions — from heavy menstrual bleeding to cancer — can now be treated with *da Vinci*® Robotic Surgery, which requires only a few small incisions.

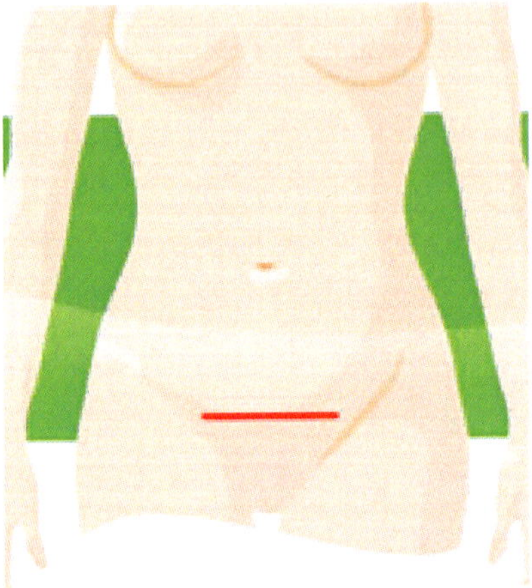

Open Surgery Incision

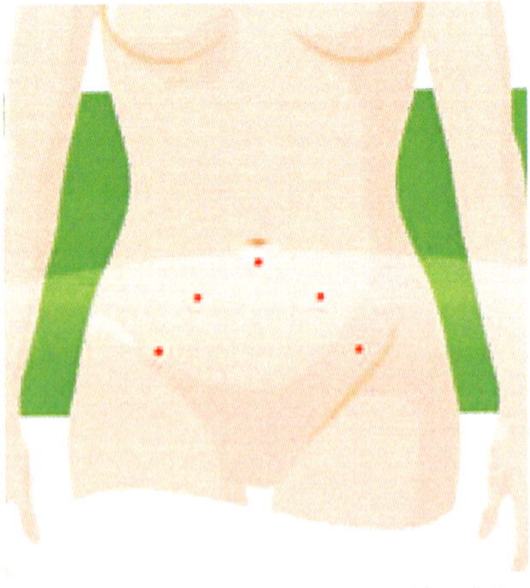

da Vinci Robotic Surgery Incisions

Need for a Hysterectomy

The most frequent reason for hysterectomy in American women is to remove fibroid tumors. These tumors account for thirty to fifty percent of the surgeries. Fibroid tumors are non-cancerous (benign) growths in the uterus that can cause pelvic and low back pain, and heavy, painful, or lengthy menstrual periods.

Twenty percent of hysterectomies are done because of abnormal vaginal bleeding that cannot be linked to any specific cause and cannot be controlled by other means. Another 20% are performed to treat prolapsed uterus, pelvic inflammatory disease, or endometrial hyperplasia, a potentially pre-cancerous condition. About 10% of hysterectomies are performed to treat cancer of the cervix, ovaries, or uterus. Women with cancer in one or more of these organs often need to have them removed as part of their cancer treatment.

Gynecologic Cancer and Other Conditions

Gynecologic cancers which are treated surgically include endometrial, ovarian, and cervical cancer. In women with endometrial cancer (a cancer of the inner lining of the uterus), comprehensive treatment can include a hysterectomy with surgical staging that includes removal of lymph nodes in the pelvis and near the aorta. Similar treatment is often recommended for women with ovarian cancer. Women with cervical cancer can benefit from a procedure called a radical hysterectomy, in which the uterus, cervix and nearby tissues are surgically removed.

Other gynecologic conditions, which most commonly require surgical correction, include symptomatic uterine fibroids, adenomyosis, endometriosis, dysmenorrhea (painful periods), and menorrhagia (excessive bleeding). In the past, these surgical procedures were performed via large abdominal incisions, also known as "open surgery" that is commonly associated with longer post-surgical recovery, increased surgical incision pain and blood loss. This often forces the woman to curtail her normal activities for several weeks.

There are Four Different Ways to Perform a Hysterectomy:

- Vaginal
- Abdominal, open or traditional
- Laparoscopy
- Robotic-assisted surgery

Vaginal

Vaginal approaches to surgery are available for some types of medical conditions, such as prolapse and menorraghia, but are not acceptable for others, such as ovarian, cervical, or advanced endometrial cancers. Vaginal approaches offer limited surgical access to the pelvic organs, and are often associated with increased vaginal pain due to the traction placed on the pelvic muscles in order to expose the organs.

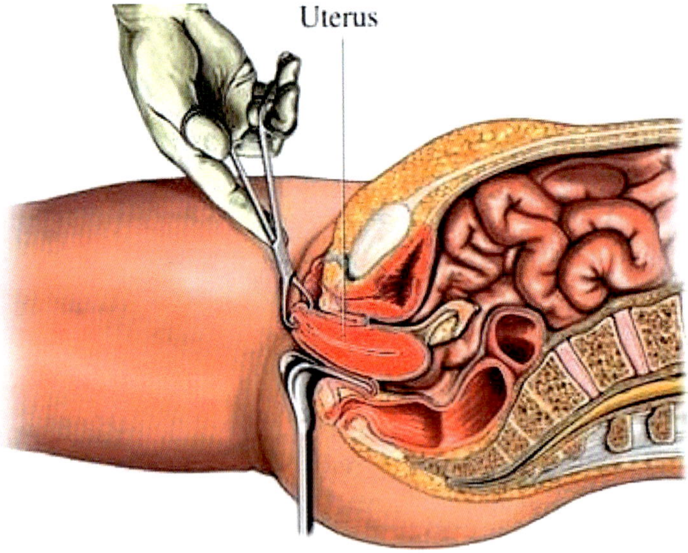

Vaginal Hysterectomy

This hysterectomy method uses a small incision inside the vagina to remove the uterus and sometimes the ovaries, as determined by your doctor. This incision is not visible externally. Vaginal hysterectomies usually require a one to three-day hospital stay and up to four weeks of recovery time.

Abdominal, Open or Traditional Method

The abdominal hysterectomy method requires a four to eight-inch horizontal incision below the belly button to remove the uterus and cervix and, in some cases, other organs. The most invasive kind of hysterectomy, this type is performed under general anesthesia, with a typical hospital stay of three to six days and up to six weeks of recovery time.

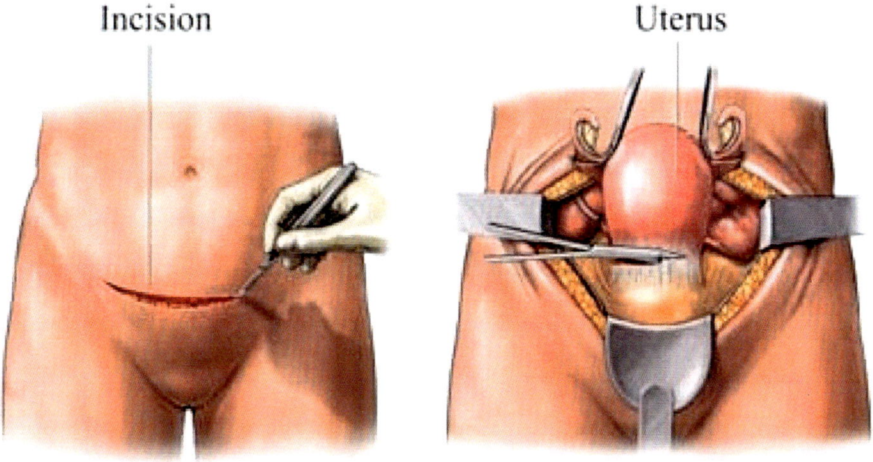

Abdominal, Open, or Traditional Hysterectomy

When faced with traditional open surgery, many women feel significant anxiety. They fear the pain and extended time for full recovery, plus the unsightly scars. For many women, their jobs and home life are deeply affected by having traditional surgery to correct a gynecologic condition, aside from the pain.

Laparoscopy

With the advent of minimally invasive surgery, a skilled surgeon can get full access to the pelvic organs by using tiny abdominal incisions. With this hysterectomy method, a thin, lighted, telescope-like instrument called a laparoscope, along with small surgical instruments, are inserted through three to four tiny incisions in the navel and abdomen to detach and remove the uterus. There are different types of laparoscopic hysterectomies. Based upon the clinical need, your doctor might perform a laparoscopic supracervical hysterectomy (LSH), allowing you to keep your cervix, or a total laparoscopic hysterectomy (TLH). Unlike more traditional methods, laparoscopic hysterectomy usually requires only one day or less in the hospital and only a few days of recovery time. Patients also experience less scarring and pain compared to other hysterectomy methods.

Standard laparoscopy, the forerunner to the *da Vinci* Robotic system, affords a minimally invasive approach to hysterectomy, but limits the surgeon's ability to completely control the surgical field during the procedure.

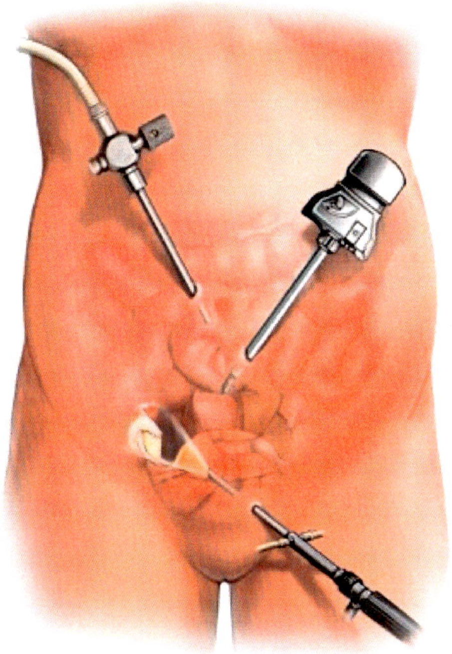

Laparoscopy

Difficulty of Laparoscopy

A doctor wrote the following to describe the difficulty of performing a laparoscopy:

Imagine waking and going through your morning rituals. Your eyes provide guidance to you as you brush your teeth. With a right and left eye, you are able to appreciate depth as you place the toothpaste on the toothbrush. Your hands and wrists work together, coordinating fine movements to grasp the toothbrush as you begin brushing.

Now, imagine going through this ritual with one eye closed and your hands are replaced with paws. You are no longer able to perceive depth. The toothpaste hits the sink, missing its intended target.

You are unable to grasp the toothbrush and your awkward movements render the complex task of brushing your teeth impossible.

Traditional laparoscopy provides this two dimensional view of the operating field. The instruments used in traditional laparoscopy act as paws, able to move only in and out, right and left.

Advantages of Robotic Surgery

A robotic surgical procedure surpasses the limits of conventional laparoscopic surgery by permitting the surgeon to have complete control of the surgical field, with natural three-dimensional vision, and wristed instruments that mimic the gross and fine movements of the human hand and fingers. Unlike laparoscopy, the surgeon regains the benefits found with open surgery. The surgeon can operate the instruments through tiny incisions, with real life visualization. This combination offers a dramatic improvement in the surgeon's ability to see and handle tissues in a way that may allow for improved surgical outcomes.

The *da Vinci* Surgical System is revolutionizing hysterectomies for women. Since the robotic gynecologic procedures were cleared by the FDA in 2005, surgeons have performed more than 200,000 *da Vinci* hysterectomies. Because of improved visualization, manipulation, and access, the *da Vinci* Surgical System permits surgeons to deal with more complex uterine pathology, such as large fibroid uteruses and dense scar tissue, by using minimally invasive techniques, rather than having to make a large incision.

The robotic system is designed to make gynecological surgery more effective and safe for the patient and more comfortable for the surgeon. It is certainly the most advanced surgical method available today.

Benefits to Patients

Reports of faster recovery, quicker return to work, decreased blood loss and less surgical pain are common among women who have undergone a robotic hysterectomy.

With complex hysterectomies and other gynecologic procedures, such as prolapse surgery, the *da Vinci* Robotic Surgical System affords women the most effective, least invasive treatment option currently available.

Comparative Costs

Many people believe that laparoscopic and robotic surgeries are more expensive than traditional or open surgery. This may be true for the cost of the actual surgery. However, a less invasive surgery, such as robotic Surgery, decreases costs outside the operating room. There are fewer costs attributed to lab work, hospital room and board, complications, infections and nursing.

There is also a significant financial advantage to patients because they return home sooner. Women who work outside the home can return to work within a week or two, compared with four to six weeks for open surgery. Taking into account the cost of the entire hospital stay and the shorter time away from work, minimally invasive surgery is less expensive than open surgery and robotic surgery is arguably equivalent, in effect and surgical outcome, to open surgery.

2

Understanding the da Vinci® Robotic Surgical System

SURGICAL MANAGEMENT USING ROBOTIC procedures is at a new level of efficiency and precision. The surgeon can perform complex maneuvers through incisions that are only one centimeter wide. Most patients are hospitalized for less than twenty-four hours, which is half of what is required following conventional open surgery.

For women facing gynecologic surgery, the period of discomfort, and extended time away from daily activities that usually follows traditional open surgery, can understandably cause significant anxiety. Fortunately, less invasive options are available. For complex problems like large fibroids, enlarged uterus, dense scar tissue, advanced cancers, endometriosis, and complex prolapse, the *da Vinci* Robotic Surgical System is undoubtedly the most effective, minimally invasive treatment option available today. Through tiny incisions, surgeons using the *da Vinci* Surgical System can operate with greater precision and control and minimize the pain, blood loss, and risk associated with large incisions.

Robotic Technology

Robotic surgery transforms laparoscopic surgery (the forerunner to the robotic system) by providing a realistic, high definition, three-dimensional view with "zoom" capability, and "wristed" instruments. These instruments have tips that mimic the intricate movements of the human hand and allow the surgeon to view the operative field in great detail, and, in turn, manipulate the instruments in the same way that their hands and fingers would move with open surgery.

This new technology gives surgeons greater visualization. The high definition, 3D camera projects images to the surgeon, who is seated at a console. The surgeon's three-dimensional view of the patient's anatomy allows for greater magnification (zooming) and offers the ability to see tissues and organs in great detail, improving surgical precision.

Comfort and Control for the Surgeon

While performing the surgical procedure with the *da Vinci* technology, the surgeon is seated at a console close to the patient. Instead of relying on an assistant to control the camera, the surgeon maintains complete control of the camera and up to three wristed laparoscopic instruments simultaneously. The surgeon can operate with equal efficiency from either side of the patient.

Many surgeons report increased ergonomic comfort while performing surgery with the *da Vinci* Robotic Surgical System. They experience less of the fatigue that is usually associated with non-robotic surgery. Less fatigue and more comfort for the surgeon result in better concentration and ability to focus on the surgical procedure with minimized distractions. In the hands of a skilled surgeon, this arrangement allows for improved surgical control and better outcomes for patients.

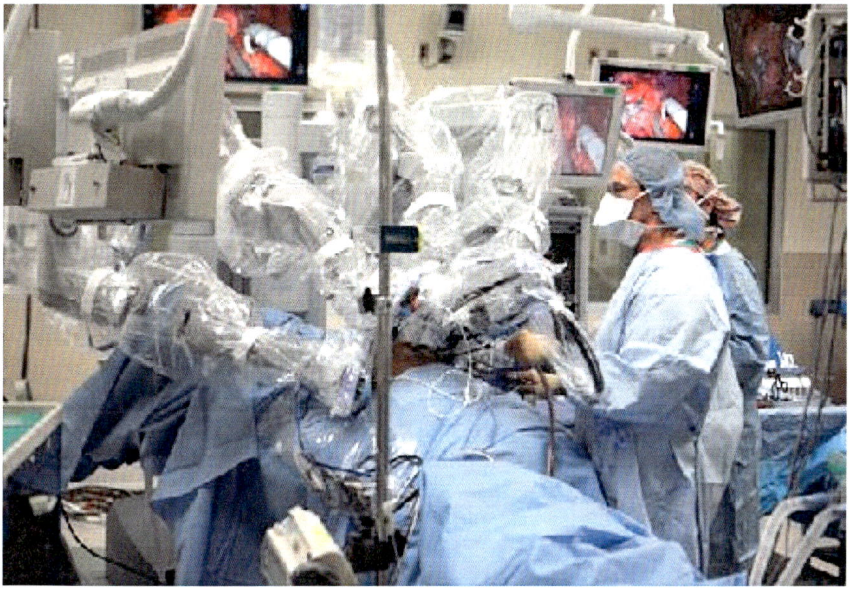

Operating Room during the Robotic Surgical Procedure

©2010 Lennox Hoyte MD.

Comparisons Between Laparoscopy and Robotic Surgery

The *da Vinci* Robotic Surgery System takes laparoscopic surgery to a higher level. The key elements in laparoscopic surgery include a laparoscope that consists of a telescopic rod lens system, usually connected to a video camera. The camera is usually placed into a one-centimeter laparoscopic port at, or near, the umbilicus (belly button). Up to three additional laparoscopic ports are put in place in the abdomen to allow placement of rod-like surgical instruments that are used to carry out the surgical procedure.

Then, harmless carbon dioxide gas is placed into the abdominal cavity in order to distend (expand) the abdomen, so that the organs and tissues can be viewed and manipulated with the instruments. The carbon dioxide gas is removed from the abdominal cavity at the end of the surgical procedure.

In laparoscopy, the surgeon usually controls only two of the instruments. The camera and the other laparoscopic instrument are most often operated by a bedside surgical assistant. The outcome of the surgery is heavily dependent on the skill of the surgeon as well as that of the assistant.

Similarly, with the *da Vinci* Robotic System, the ports are placed (though in slightly different positions than for laparoscopy) and the abdomen is distended with carbon dioxide gas. In robotic surgery, the ports are then attached to robotic arms. These instruments have substantially greater flexibility than the laparoscopic instruments, and the surgeon maintains direct control of the camera and three of the instruments. In addition, the 3D visualization with zoom capability dramatically improves the surgeon's perception of the tissues, leading to greater surgical precision. A single assistant port allows for passage of sutures into the surgical field and also for the removal of specimens.

The da Vinci 3D Optics

The *da Vinci* Robotic Surgical System is made up of many technologically advanced parts, including a sophisticated stereoscopic digital camera.

The camera consists of two high definition units. Much like human eyes, these cameras recreate a true 3D color image which is viewed by the surgeon at the console. The images are clearly visible and provide the surgeon with depth perception while performing the procedure. The camera allows for up to 12x magnification of the field, opening up the possibility of performing microsurgical procedures on the urinary and fallopian tubes, as well as spotting and managing small blood vessels to reduce the risk of surgical bleeding.

This "Insite-Vision" System is one of the most advanced vision systems available today.

During surgery, the camera is held by a central robotic arm that is connected to one of the laparoscopy ports. The camera provides stereoscopic visualization, and lighting into the abdomen, illuminating the tissues and organs of interest to the surgeon. The surgeon controls the robotic arms (including the camera arm) from the console.

Greater Precision

Through tiny incisions, surgeons using the *da Vinci* System can operate with greater precision and minimize the pain, blood loss, and risk associated with large incisions.

Robotic surgery transforms laparoscopic surgery by providing a realistic, high definition, three-dimensional view with "zoom" capability, and "wristed" instruments with tips that mimic the intricate movements of the human hand. These elements allow the surgeon to view the operative field in great detail, and in turn manipulate the instruments in the same way that their hands and fingers would move during open surgery.

This new technology has given the skilled surgeon greater visualization with a high definition, 3D camera projecting images to the surgeon seated at a console. The surgeon's three-dimensional view of the patient's anatomy allows for greater magnification, and offers the ability to see tissues and organs in great detail, improving surgical precision. Also, rather than depending on an assistant to manage the camera and other instruments, which has been the method in the past, the *da Vi*nci surgeon maintains complete control of the camera and up to three wristed robotic instruments simultaneously while performing the surgical procedure. The surgeon controls these instruments from a surgical console placed near the patient. Surgeons report increased ergonomic comfort. Comfort translates into a less distracted surgeon who is better able to concentrate on the surgical field.

Understanding Robotic Surgery

In order to understand robotic surgery, an understanding of traditional laparoscopy is needed. The key element in laparoscopic surgery is a laparoscope that consists of a telescopic rod lens system, usually connected to a video camera. Additional laparoscopic ports are put in place in the abdomen to allow placement of rod-like surgical instruments, which are used to carry out the surgical procedure. In addition, carbon dioxide is placed into the abdominal cavity in order to distend the abdomen, so that the organs and tissues can be viewed through the laparoscopic camera. The pelvic organs and tissues are manipulated via instruments placed in the additional ports. The surgeon usually operates two of the laparoscopic instruments, and the camera and other laparoscopic instruments are most often operated by a bedside assistant. The carbon dioxide gas is removed from the abdominal cavity at the end of the surgical procedure. The outcome of the surgery is heavily dependent on the skill of the surgeon, as well as that of the bedside assistant.

Many aspects of *da Vinci* surgery are similar to traditional laparoscopy. However, with the *da Vinci* Robotic Surgical System, the instruments have substantially greater flexibility, and the surgeon maintains control of the camera and three of the instruments. In addition, the 3D visualization dramatically improves surgeon perception of the tissues, leading to greater surgical precision. A single assistant port allows for passage of sutures into the surgical field, and also for the removal of specimens.

During surgery, the *da Vinci* Robotic Surgical System has the surgeon seated at a console where he/she can perform the surgery in an ergonomically comfortable environment, close to the patient.

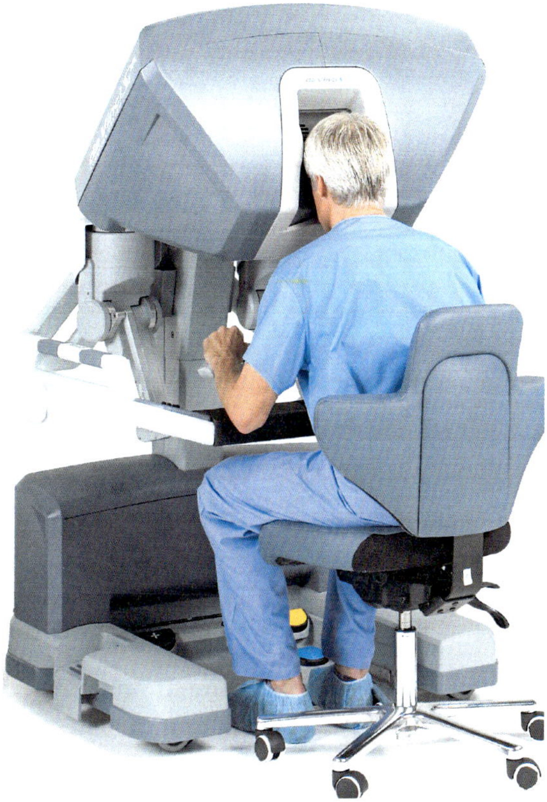

Surgeon at the da Vinci Robotic Console

The Cameras

During surgery, the camera is held by a central robotic arm that is connected to one of the laparoscopy ports. The camera provides stereoscopic visualization and lighting into the abdomen, illuminating the tissues and organs of interest to the surgeon. The surgeon controls the robotic arms (including the camera arm) from the console.

Three cameras are available for use on the *da Vinci* system. The surgeon may choose to use a straight camera, or one of two angled cameras. The straight camera is used for viewing tissues that are directly in front of the camera itself. The angled cameras come in two types, an "up" pointing type, and a "down" pointing type.

The up and down cameras can be used to view tissues that lie at a sharp angle from the axis of the camera port. These oblique cameras give the surgeon the freedom to view around the curved areas inside the abdomen and underneath the uterus. The optical system provides high resolution and excellent depth perception. With a sharp, clear picture, and articulating "wristed" instruments, these tools allow the surgeon to achieve a better surgical performance than with "straight stick" instruments.

The surgical instruments and a stereoscopic video camera and light source all work in unison during surgery. The hand-like surgical instruments move with seven degrees of freedom and two degrees of axial rotation. The ten-millimeter video telescope contains two separate five-millimeter telescopes that are attached to two separate three-chip video cameras. The offset of the two telescopes permit a telecast of a true three-dimensional image through the binocular imaging system. The surgeon sees a three-dimensional virtual operative field.

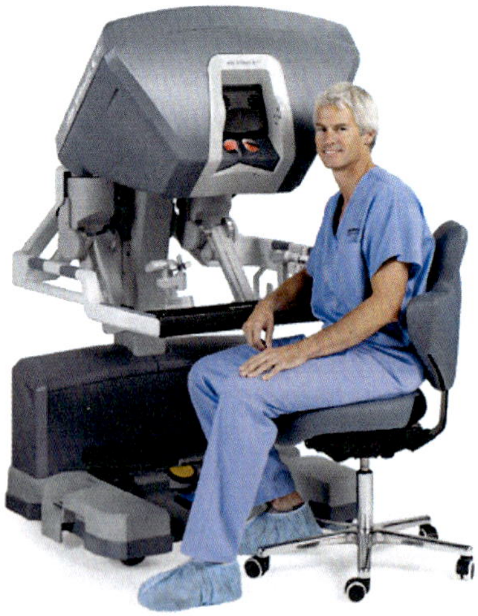

View of the Console

©2010 Intuitive Surgical, Inc.

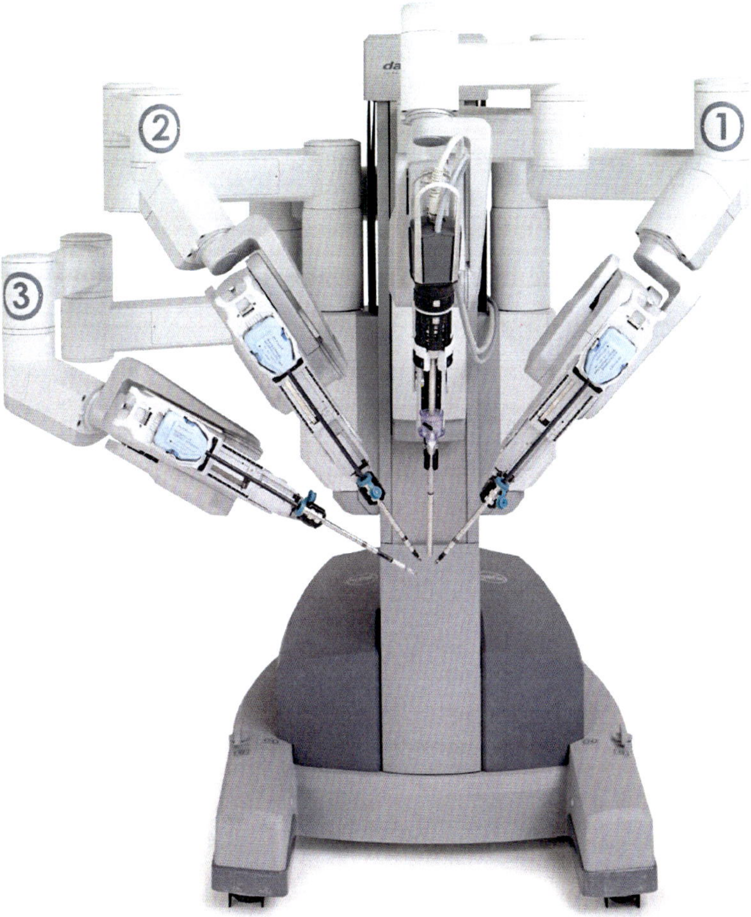

da Vinci Patient Cart - front with instruments

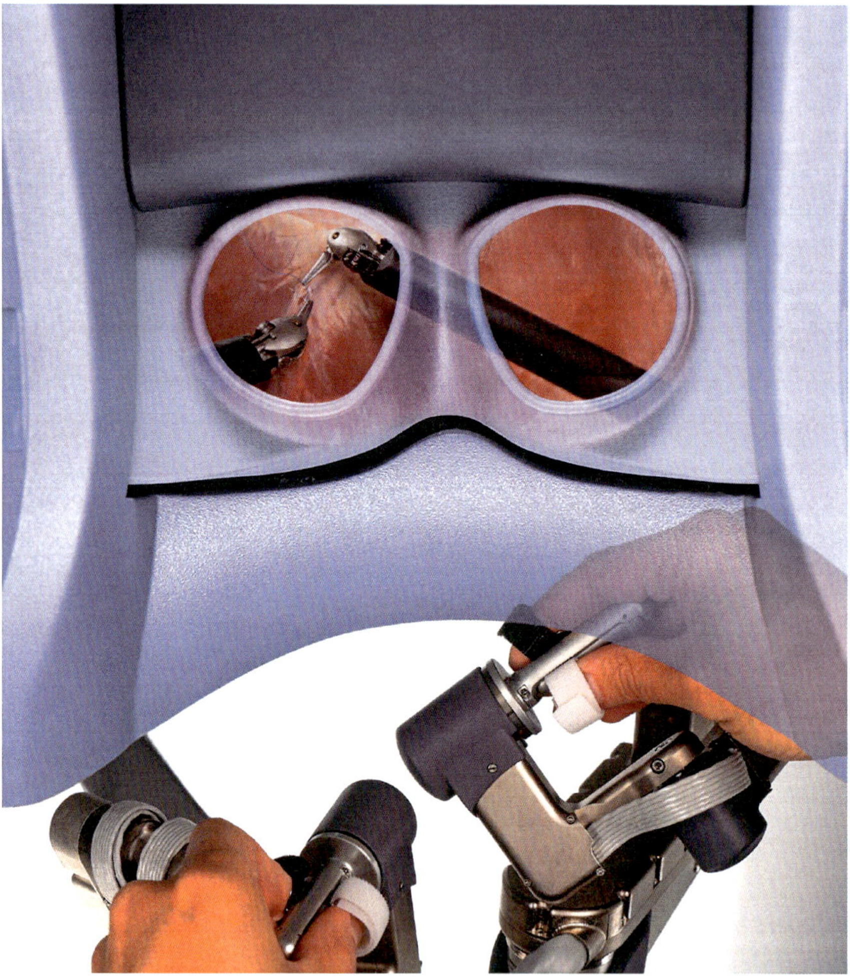

The High Resolution, High Frame-Rate Eyepieces for ViewingEndoscopic Pictures of Nearly 12 x Magnification.

Full Range of Hand Motion

Unlike laparoscopic approach, the *da Vinci* robotic instrumentation provides surgeons with a full range of motion, and the patient loses significantly less blood. For this reason, robotic-assisted surgery is sometimes called bloodless surgery.

By replicating the surgeon's hand movements, there is greater dexterity than that of the surgeon's wrists and fingers. Notice in the photo, the range of motion and ability of the robotic hand to twist and turn with greater ability than the human hand. It is important to note that all movements of the robotic hand are controlled by the surgeon offering precise motions on command.

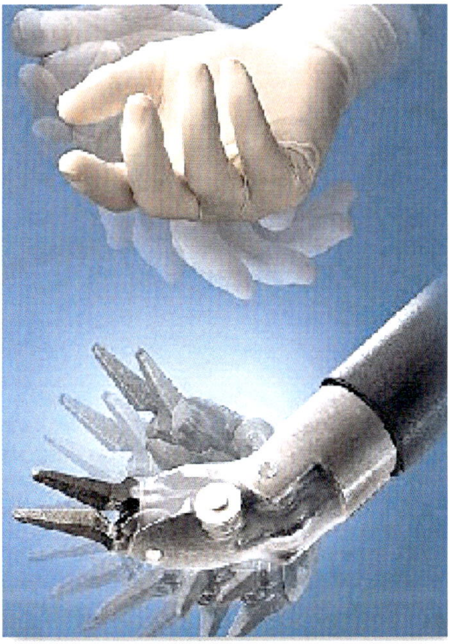

The proprietary *EndoWrist®* Instruments, powered by state-of-the-art robotic technology, offer hand movements that are scaled, filtered and seamlessly translated into precise movements of the *EndoWrist* Instruments. The EndoWrist has greater use of "fingers" than the human hand.

da Vinci Si

During surgery, the surgeon seated at the console can look through what appears to be binoculars inset in the console and views the magnified, three-dimensional surgical field. The surgeon's fingers and thumb are placed in the ring finger of each hand with plastic loops below the console.

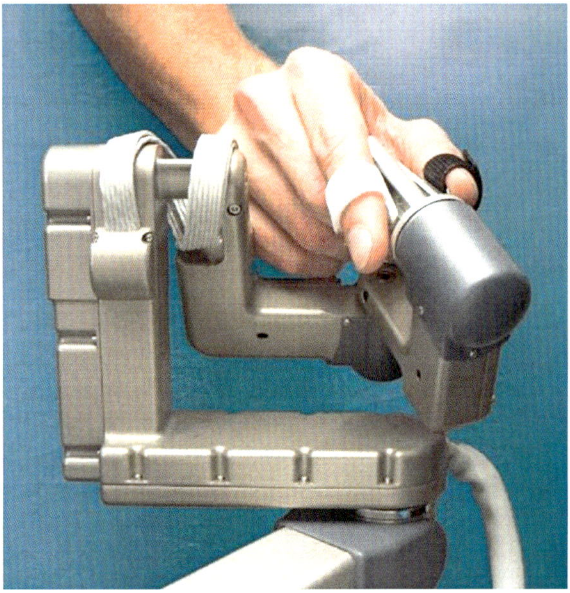

Hand Movement Instruments are Finger Locked In.

da Vinci Si

Robotic Hand

Specialized technology transfers the surgeon's exact hand movements at the console to the extremely precise micro-surgical movements of the robotic instruments ("hands") inside the patient's abdomen. Instruments include different kinds of forceps (grasping instruments, similar to tweezers), scissors, suture needle drivers, and other types of grasping and cutting instruments. Through the incisions, the surgeon can rotate the instruments 360 degrees.

The *da Vinci* system also allows for the removal of natural tremors from the hands of the surgeon. The system allows for control of the coarseness or fine-ness of the movements transmitted to the instruments. In effect, the system can magnify or shrink the surgeon's hand movements, depending on the chosen settings. Tremors, though very slight, are part of every human hand. The *da Vinci* system eliminates these tremors.

The *da Vinci* surgical instruments are, at first glance, similar to standard laparoscopic instruments. However, the *da Vinci* surgical instruments have an advantage: they can be articulated. This gives the instruments not only the ability to open and close, but to fully turn and twist. These surgical instruments are designed with jointed wrists, which provide freedom of movement in multiple directions known as "seven degrees of freedom."

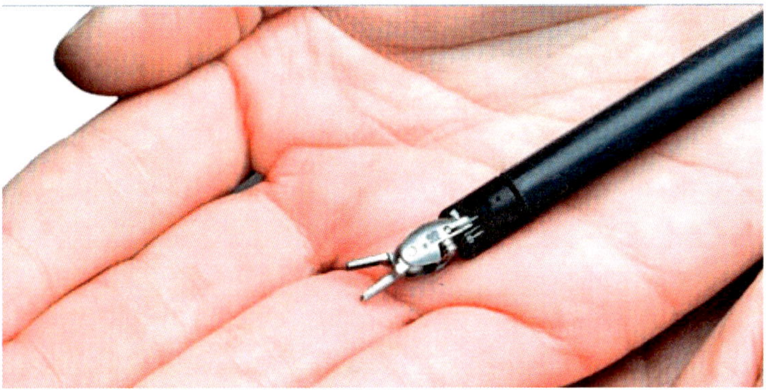

The da Vinci System's Small Hand-Movement Tools

da Vinci Si

It is as if a human hand were twisting and turning in motion. Yet, unlike the surgeon's hand, these instruments are considerably smaller. Some of the "jaws" of the tools are similar in size to, and with some, shorter in length than a fingernail. These amazingly accurate and tiny instruments empower the surgeon with extremely fine coordination and accuracy.

Computerized da Vinci System Arms

The computerized *da Vinci* system also consists of a four-arm robot that is controlled by the surgeon at the console — the command center of the procedure offering precision surgery. The arms of the instrument can hold and manipulate a host of items simultaneously, including the camera and several highly refined surgical instruments. One surgeon said this of the robotic arms: "It gives the surgeon another pair of arms to work with; it's like having four arms working simultaneously."

Traditional Instruments Versus da Vinci Surgical Instruments

Standard "straight stick" laparoscopic instruments are manipulated counter-intuitively or 'backwards.' This means that, with laparoscopy, the surgeon's hand motions need to be opposite of what the surgeon wishes the instrument tip to do. To move the instrument tip to the right, the surgeon must move the handle to the left, and vice versa. To move the tip up, the surgeon must move the handle down. This requires a laparoscopic surgeon to "think opposite," or move in mirror image to the way that the instrument should go.

The robotic surgical system removes these limitations. The instruments move in the same direction as the surgeon's hands. If the surgeon turns left, the robotic instrument turns left, up or down, right or left, motion is the same as the surgeon's hand operating it.

Also, because the instrument movements can be scaled down, the surgeon at the console can make micro precise dissections with these mechanical movements.

Studies have also revealed that the robotic system reduces surgeon fatigue (which inevitably occurs when surgery lasts more than an hour) due to the fact that the surgeon is manipulating the instruments seated in favorable position with little force on the hand.

Console, Surgical Cart and the Connection Between the Two

The surgical cart is located beside the patient and utilizes one robotic arm to control the endoscope (which provides stereoscopic or 3-D vision) and three robotic arms to control the surgical instruments.

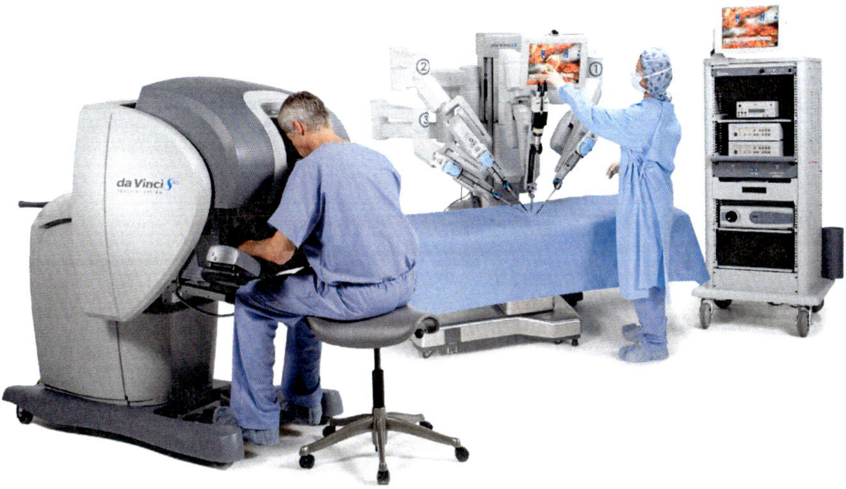

da Vinci Setup of Instruments

da Vinci Si

How Robot-Assisted Surgery Works

As with Laparoscopic Minimally Invasive Surgery (LMIS), the surgeon inserts miniature surgical instruments and a camera into small incisions in the patient. These incisions are also called ports. Unlike LMIS, the surgeon controls the movement of the instruments and camera at a robotic console in the operating room. The console is equipped with a special three-dimensional monitor and user-friendly hand controls that allow for control of the surgical instruments using natural hand movements. The Surgeon Console contains the master controls that the surgeon uses to manipulate the EndoWrist robotic Instruments.

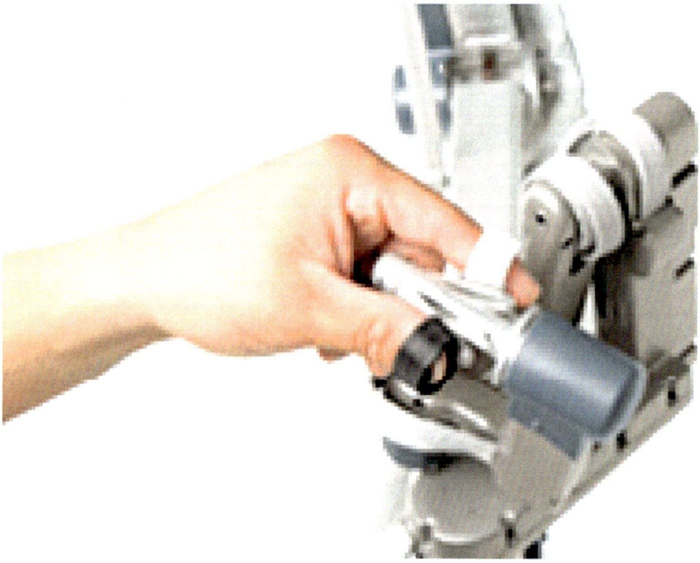

While working the EndoWrist instrument, the surgeon's fingers are placed in rings to keep the hand from inadvertently bumping the controls during surgery.

da Vinci Si

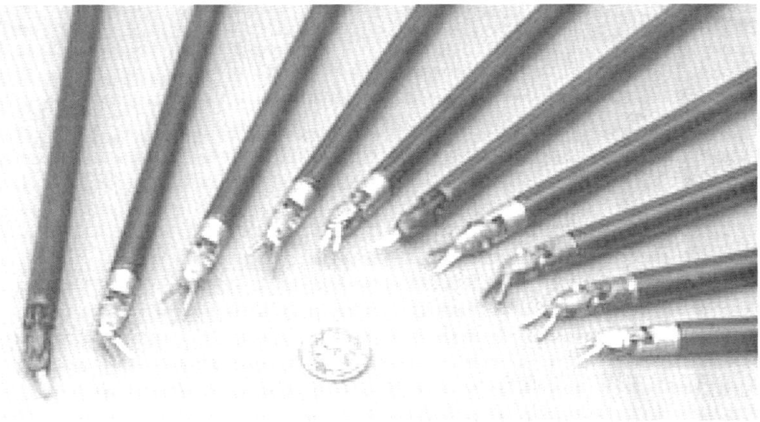

The specialized technology of the da Vinci System transfers the surgeon's exact hand movements at the console to the extremely precise micro-surgical movements of the three robotic pincers ("hands") inside the patient's body. The surgeon can rotate the instruments 360 degrees through the incisions.

da Vinci Si

3

Methods of Gynecologic Surgery

WHEN MEDICATION AND NON-INVASIVE measures fail to relieve symptoms, surgery remains the accepted and most effective treatment for a range of gynecologic conditions. These include, but are not limited to, cervical, ovarian, and uterine cancer, uterine fibroids, endometriosis, painful periods, uterine prolapse and menorrhagia or excessive bleeding.

There are several methods by which the surgeon can perform an operation. These include open surgery, as well as vaginal, laparoscopic, and robotic approaches.

Open Hysterectomy

Traditionally, surgeons have performed the majority of hysterectomies using an "open" approach, which is through a large abdominal incision. An open approach to the hysterectomy procedure requires a 6-12 inch incision in the abdomen. The incision can be vertical (up and down), extending from the pubic bone, up to or at times past the belly button in the midline, or sideways (bikini cut) made just above the pubic bone, extending from one side of the lower abdomen to the other. Either way, the incision will leave a large scar in the abdomen.

The benefit of the open approach is that it provides a wide open exposure for the surgeon and access for the surgeon's hands, which allows for a direct "feel" of the tissues. Open surgery for most gynecological problems has been performed for decades. Recovery time tends to be longer and more painful with these types of incisions.

For women facing a hysterectomy, using the open technique means greater postsurgical pain, discomfort and extended time away from normal daily activities. This understandably causes significant anxiety.

Vaginal Approach

Fortunately, less invasive options are available. Some gynecologic procedures enable surgeons to access the uterus, and surgically remove it using a vaginal approach, which does not normally require an external incision.

Without an external incision, there is no subsequent abdominal scarring. Surgeons most often use this minimally invasive approach when the patient's condition is benign, or when the uterus is normal size. The vaginal approach may also be used when the condition is limited to the uterus, and when there is no anticipated need to access all of the pelvic organs. The vaginal approach allows for faster recovery than the traditional open method, yet it can still be the cause of postoperative pains.

Laparoscopic Hysterectomy

A laparoscopic approach is also an accepted method for accessing and surgically removing the uterus. With the laparoscopic approach, a small incision (called a port) is made at or near the umbilicus (belly button), and a camera and light are inserted through the port into the abdomen. The abdomen is then insufflated (filled) with carbon dioxide gas, which distends the abdomen so that the organs and tissues can be viewed optimally. Two to three additional ports are then created in the mid or lower abdomen, and the laparoscopic instruments are placed through these additional ports. The additional instruments are usually a grasping instrument (like tweezers), a cutting instrument (like scissors), and some type of suturing instrument. The instruments are used to disconnect the uterus from its internal connections, and remove it from the abdominal cavity. The method of removing the uterus depends on the type of hysterectomy performed. For the total hysterectomy, the uterus is removed through the vagina, and the opening in the vagina is closed with sutures (stitches). For the subtotal (supracervical) hysterectomy, only the top of the uterus is removed, usually by cutting it into small pieces (morcellating) and removing the pieces through one of the laparoscopic ports. If needed, the ovaries and tubes may also be removed along with the uterus, either through the vagina, or through morcellation.

Laparoscopic surgeons use this minimally invasive approach for a wide range of uterine conditions, including cancer. The laparoscopic approach works well for smaller uteruses, but may be applied to more complex uterine pathology as well, depending on the skill of the surgeon. This approach requires a very highly skilled surgical assistant who is responsible for manipulating the camera and one of the instruments, under guidance from the surgeon. For more complex pathology, the lack of 3D vision and wristed instruments can make laparoscopy exceptionally challenging especially for larger, fibroid uteruses, and procedures requiring extensive suturing (e.g., prolapse repair). This approach allows for faster recovery, yet can still be the source of postoperative pains.

Robotic Hysterectomy

For more complex hysterectomies, robot-assisted surgery may be the most effective, minimally invasive treatment option available. Examples of complex situations include those where a woman has a larger uterus, advanced cancer, dense adhesions, or requires extensive suturing (for example, in the case of advanced prolapse). Through tiny, one-centimeter incisions, robotic surgeons can operate with greater precision and control to remove the uterus, while having tightly controlled access to the entire pelvis in a reliable way. Using microsurgical techniques, surgeons can minimize the pain and risk associated with large incisions while increasing surgical access to the organs in the abdomen.

While minimally invasive vaginal and laparoscopic hysterectomies offer important potential advantages to patients over open abdominal hysterectomy – including reduced risk for complications, a shorter hospitalization and faster recovery – there are inherent drawbacks. With vaginal hysterectomy, surgeons are challenged by a small working space and a limited view of the pelvic organs.

Additional conditions can make the vaginal approach difficult, including the patient who has a very large uterus, fibroids, pelvic adhesions, and pathology requiring access to the upper abdominal organs. These factors can reduce the possibility of completing the surgery vaginally.

In laparoscopic surgery the surgeon must cope with "straight stick" instruments, which lack dexterity, and move in a direction opposite to the surgeon's hand movements. Additionally, there is a need to have a highly skilled assistant to manipulate the camera and some of the instruments. These limitations make laparoscopic suturing (stitching) extremely difficult, and limits access to deep areas in the pelvis. With laparoscopy, the surgeon can directly control only two instruments at a time.

Robotic Surgery enables gynecologic surgeons to perform the most precise, minimally invasive hysterectomy available. For most women, a robotically performed hysterectomy offers numerous potential benefits over traditional open surgery, including:

- Significantly less pain
- Minimal blood loss and need for transfusion
- Fewer complications
- Shorter hospital stay
- Quicker recovery and return to normal activities1,

- Small incisions for minimal scarring
- Better patient satisfaction, in many cases[3]

Reference

Boggess JF. Robotic surgery in gynecologic oncology: evolution of a new surgical paradigm. J Robotic Surg 2007 1:31-3[2] Payne TN, et al. A comparison of total laparoscopic hysterectomy to robotically assisted hysterectomy: surgical outcomes in a community practice. J Minim Invasive Gynecol. 2008 May-June;15(3):286-91

In a study documenting his early experiences with robotic surgery, Dr. Shashoua compared the first 27 robotic hysterectomies to the prior 44 laparoscopic hysterectomies. The study showed that both techniques can be done safely and have the benefit of a short hospital stay. As compared to laparoscopic hysterectomy, robotic hysterectomy led to a reduction in length of hospital stay and a reduced need for narcotic pain medication following surgery.

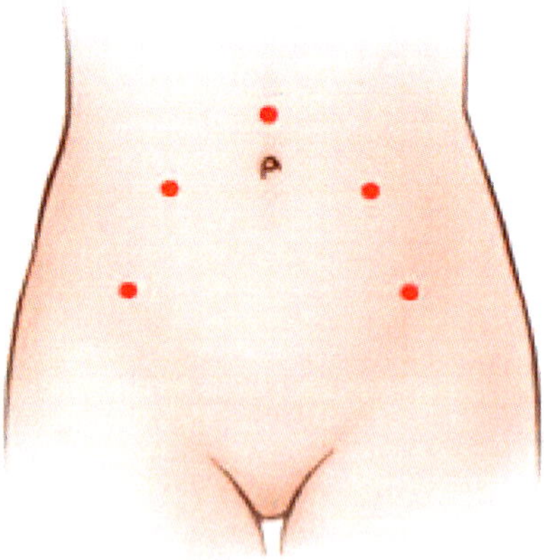

da Vinci Hysterectomy Incisions

Robotic Surgery – What the future holds:

The techniques involved in robotic surgery are constantly evolving. The next exciting frontier is Single Incision Robotic Hysterectomy. Instead of the incisions typical for robotic surgery, all instruments and camera are placed through a single incision usually hidden in the belly button. Available with the new *da Vinci* SI system, this technique is rapidly evolving. In the near future, single incision robotics may become the standard of care for hysterectomy.

Part Two

Need for Surgery

4

Female Issues that May Require A Hysterectomy

OVER 600,000 HYSTERECTOMIES ARE PERFORMED in the United States each year. The reasons for hysterectomy include cancer and pre-cancer, fibroids, excessive bleeding, painful periods, and prolapse. This chapter will go over the different reasons for undergoing hysterectomy.

Listed here are the more common female conditions that can be corrected surgically, using the robotic approach.

Gynecologic Cancers

It is a fact that breast cancer is the most common form of cancer in women. Nevertheless, more than 80,000 women in the United States alone, each year, undergo cancer surgery for uterine, cervical, and ovarian cancer. About ten percent of hysterectomies are performed to treat cancer of the cervix, ovaries, or uterus.

Uterine Cancer

In the United States, approximately 42,000 women each year are diagnosed with uterine cancer — the most common malignancy of the female genital tract and the fourth most common cancer in women.

Uterine cancer can appear in cells lining the uterus (endometrium) and in muscle or other tissues in the uterus (uterine sarcoma). Early, low-grade uterine cancer can be treated with a total hysterectomy, but advanced or high-grade uterine cancers may also require removal of the ovaries, and extensive removal of lymph nodes.

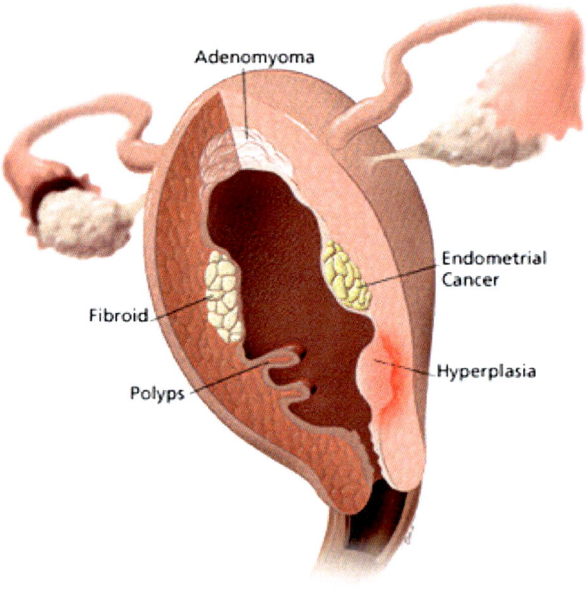

Cervical Cancer

Cervical cancer is the second most common cancer of the female reproductive system. It accounts for six percent of all cancers. The cervix is located at the neck of the uterus and connected to the upper part of the vagina. The cervix is lined with cells that normally grow, divide, shed, and are replaced on an ongoing basis. This normal growth is called mitosis and occurs throughout the body to ensure that the health and function of the cells, tissues and organ systems are maintained at optimal levels

Cervical cancer is a disease in which normal cervical lining cells are transformed into malignant (cancer) cells in the cervix. The cervix contains two types of cells that are at risk for turning cancerous. These are called the squamous cells, and glandular cells. The squamous cells line the outer part of the cervix and are the same type of cell that lines the vaginal walls. Squamous cells are the most likely to become cancerous, and these squamous cell cancers can often also involve the upper part of the vagina. Glandular cells can also become cancerous, but much less often when compared to squamous cells.

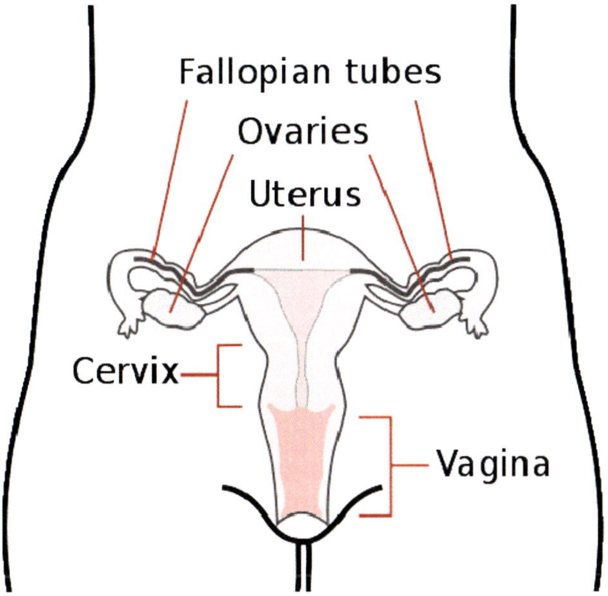

The Cervix is Located Just Above the Vagina in the Uterus

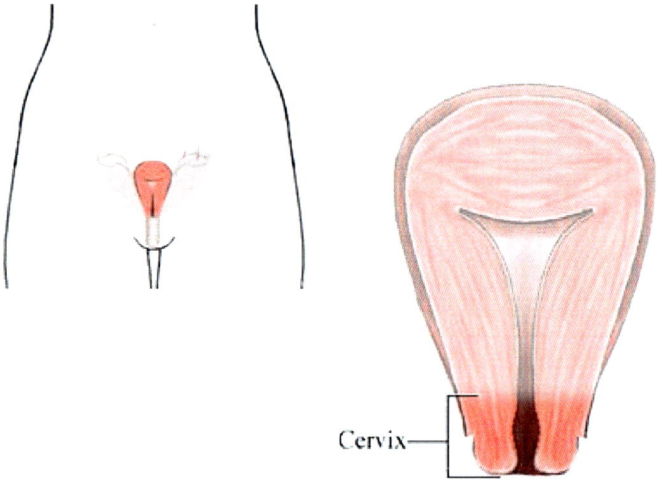

Typically, cervical cancer develops slowly over the course of several years. The cancerous cells begin to grow in the tissues of the cervix. The cervical Pap smear is designed to help locate cervical cells that may be transforming themselves into cancer. Regular Pap smear tests can detect cells that may be trying to become cancerous. When detected early, these abnormal cells can be treated with simple, noninvasive office procedures, which can completely remove the abnormal cells. However, if these abnormal cells are allowed to progress to cancer, a woman may require more invasive treatment, which can include removal of the inner part of the cervix (cervical conization), total or radical hysterectomy, and/or pelvic radiation, depending on the extent of the spread of the cancer.

Ovarian Cancer

The ovaries are a pair of walnut-sized organs in a woman's pelvic area. They are located on either side of the uterus (the organ that holds the baby when a woman is pregnant). Ovaries make and release the eggs which, when combined with a man's sperm, can grow into a baby. The ovaries also make the female hormones progesterone and estrogen, as well as small amounts of androgenic (or male) hormones. Ovarian hormones regulate the menstrual cycle, and also aid in the development and maintenance of body appearance and functions specific to women.

As with cervical cancer, ovarian cancer occurs when cells in the ovary begin changing and multiplying out of control. These cells can form lumps of tissue called tumors. Cancer that starts in the ovaries is called ovarian cancer. Ovarian cancer can spread from the ovaries to other parts of the body. This spread is called metastasis. The more cancer spreads, the harder it is to treat. Unlike endometrial cancer, which can announce its presence by abnormal bleeding, or cervical cancer, which can be detected very early with regular Pap smears; ovarian cancer can develop silently within the pelvis over a period of time. Symptoms tend to be vague, so that most ovarian cancers are harder to treat, because they are found at a more advanced stage than cervical or endometrial cancers.

Different Types of Ovarian Tumors

- Epithelial tumors form in the cells that cover the outer surface of the ovaries. This is the most common type of ovarian cancer.
- Germ cell tumors form in the cells inside the ovary that produce eggs. These rare tumors are most common in women in their teens and early twenties.
- Stromal tumors grow from the cells that make female hormones. This is one of the least common forms of ovarian cancer

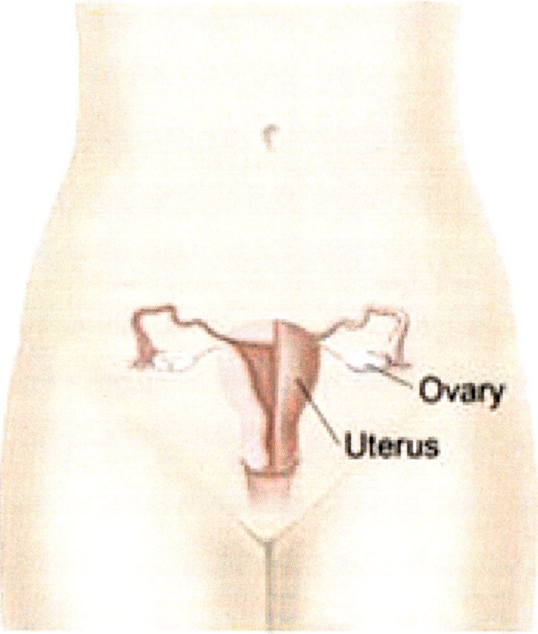

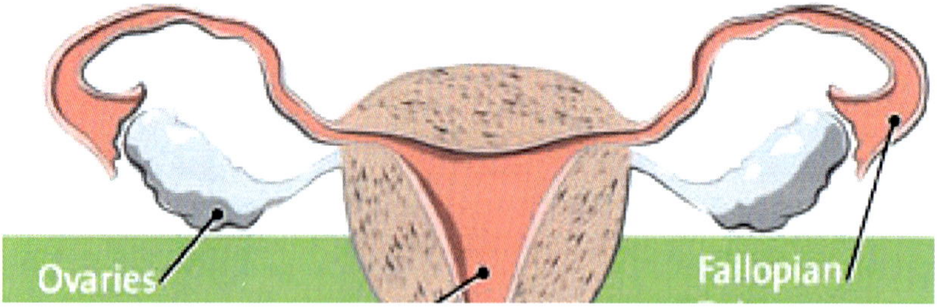

Ovaries are Located on Either Side of the Uterus.

Treatment Options for Ovarian Cancer

Treatment options for ovarian cancer may include:

- Surgery to remove the ovaries and surrounding tissues, and often the uterus.
- Chemotherapy, which uses strong medications to kill cancer cells. This treatment is often used along with surgery.

Surgery, often followed by chemotherapy is probably the most recommended treatment for ovarian cancer.

Fibroid Tumors

Fibroid tumors are non-cancerous (benign) growths in the uterus that can cause pelvic and low back pain, heavy or lengthy menstrual periods and bowel and bladder problems. Fibroid tumors may be treated by removing the fibroids (myomectomy) or, if a woman does not desire future fertility, hysterectomy. Some fibroids grow on the outside layer of the uterus (subserosal fibroids), others grow along the inner lining of the uterus (sub mucosal fibroids), and still others grow within the muscular wall of the uterus (intramural fibroids). A third of all hysterectomies are performed to treat fibroids.

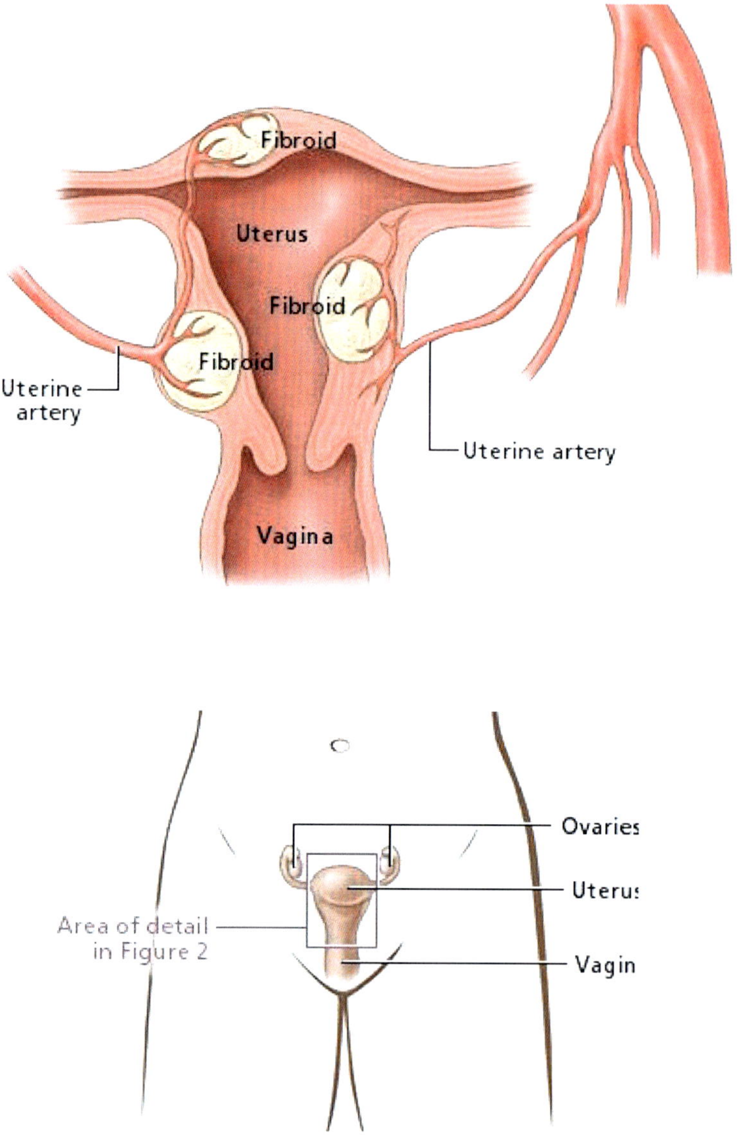

Anatomy of Uterine Fibroids

Abnormal Vaginal Bleeding

When irregular vaginal bleeding occurs in the absence of fibroids, cancer, and damage to the vagina or any other anatomic abnormality, this is called dysfunctional bleeding or abnormal vaginal bleeding. The first line of therapy is the use of medications and uterine inserts to regulate the bleeding. When these fail, therapies like dilation and curettage (D&C) to scrape the uterine lining, or endometrial ablation to destroy the inner lining of the uterus may be recommended. If these procedures fail to stop the bleeding, a hysterectomy may be recommended. Twenty percent of all hysterectomies are performed to relieve abnormal vaginal bleeding.

Prolapse, Pelvic Inflammatory Disease and Endometrial Hyperplasia

Prolapsed uterus and vagina, pelvic inflammatory disease, and endometrial hyperplasia, together account for twenty percent of hysterectomies.

Prolapse

Pelvic organ prolapse (including cystocele, rectocele, enterocele, and proccidentia) occurs when the support for the uterus and vaginal tissues is lost, causing the vagina to turn "inside out", often leading to a vaginal bulge, pelvic pressure, and low back pain. Prolapse often happens due to childbirth followed by aging, or sometimes following hysterectomy. But some women who never delivered a baby can develop prolapse. In women with a uterus, hysterectomy with vaginal vault resuspension is the definitive surgical treatment for this condition.

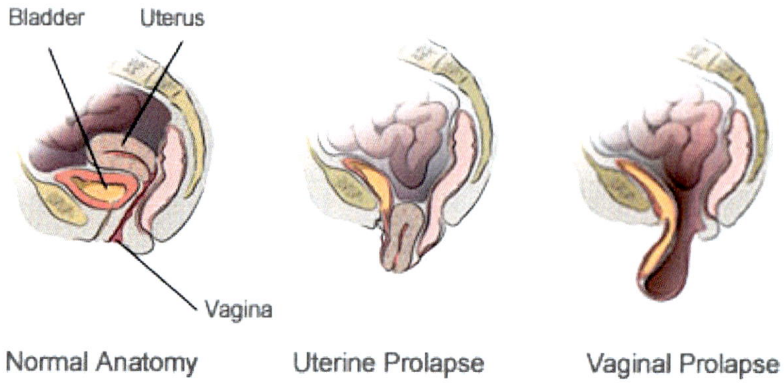

Pelvic Inflammatory Disease
Pelvic inflammatory disease is an advanced infection in the uterus or tubes. Early diagnosis of pelvic inflammatory disease, and aggressive treatment with antibiotics can decrease the need for hysterectomy to treat this condition.

Endometrial Hyperplasia Endometrial hyperplasia is a potentially pre-cancerous condition that can cause irregular bleeding, but is also treatable with medication and less dramatic procedures like dilation and curettage (D&C), in which the uterine lining is surgically scraped to remove the abnormal endometrial tissue, and cure the bleeding problem. There can sometimes be cancer cells hidden among the hyperplasia. If these are found at the time of D&C, appropriate treatment for endometrial cancer is recommended.

Adenomyosis

In this condition, the tissue that lines the uterus grows inside the walls of the uterus, which can cause severe pain, and sometimes pain with sexual intercourse. Nonsurgical therapies include stopping or regulating the menstrual cycle with medications. If these treatments fail to control the symptoms, and the woman does not desire future fertility, a hysterectomy may be effective in curing the painful symptoms.

Chronic Pelvic Pain

Many women with chronic pelvic pain may be treated non-surgically, with anti-inflammatory medications, biofeedback, and/or physical therapy. When these and other non-surgical therapies fail to cure the symptoms, a hysterectomy may be the last resort for women who have chronic pelvic pain that clearly comes from the uterus. Unfortunately, for many women with symptoms of chronic pelvic pain, a hysterectomy will not cure the pain symptom, and may create new sources of pain.

5

Candidates for a Hysterectomy

ONLY A WOMAN AND HER doctor can decide whether hysterectomy is right for her. Once the decision for hysterectomy is made, the woman and her surgeon should consider if Robotic Surgery is right for her. Before making the decision, the patient should make sure she is aware of all the surgical options available, as well as the physician's experience and skill as a robotic surgeon.

A patient, to determine if she is a candidate for *da Vin*ci Robotic Surgery, must get the information needed from a consultation with a qualified, experienced surgeon. In order to better understand their choices with regards to hysterectomy, patients need to gain a basic knowledge of the female reproductive anatomy, and also understand the types of conditions which may be treated with hysterectomy.

Female Reproductive System Anatomy

The female reproductive system consists of the uterus and cervix, ovaries, and fallopian tubes. The uterus is a hollow, muscular organ that holds a baby as it grows inside a pregnant woman. The fallopian tubes and ovaries are located on either side of the uterus. The ovaries supply the eggs, which may be fertilized by a man's sperm to become a fetus growing in the uterus.

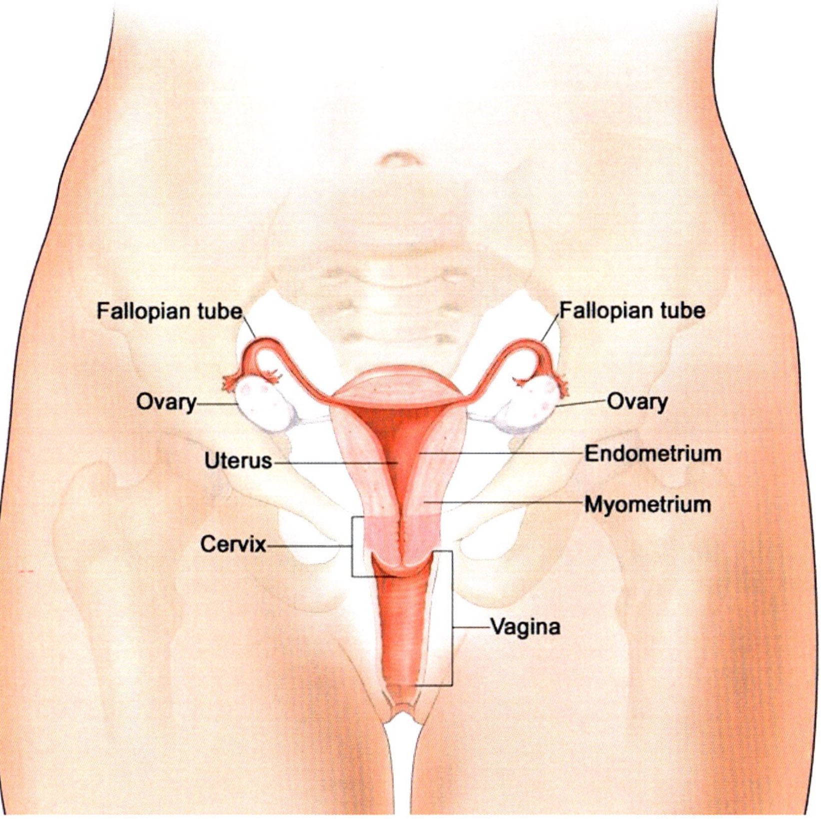

The female reproductive system

The fallopian tubes provide a pathway for the eggs to reach the uterus to become fertilized and implant into the lining of the uterus. The lining of the uterus is called the endometrium, and this tissue grows, sheds, and re-grows each month during a woman's reproductive years. The lymph nodes are tiny pea sized organs that the body uses to collect and destroy harmful substances like cancer cells, and some infectious agents. Each organ has a set of associated lymph nodes, which are positioned around the blood vessels that supply and drain blood from that organ. If an organ becomes cancerous, cells from the cancer can sometimes spread to the nearby lymph nodes.

The ovaries, cervix, and fallopian tubes also undergo monthly changes during reproductive years. These regular changes put these tissues at increased risk for malignancy or cancer. The most common types of gynecologic cancers are cervical, endometrial (uterine), and ovarian cancer. The specific type of cancer a woman has, and how advanced it is, will determine her available treatment options.

Conditions treatable with a Hysterectomy

Common conditions that may be treated with hysterectomy include reproductive system cancers, abnormal uterine bleeding, certain types of pelvic pain, pelvic organ prolapse, and symptomatic fibroids. Reproductive system cancers include endometrial (uterine), cervical, ovarian, and fallopian tube cancers.

Gynecologic Cancers

Women with gynecologic cancers are often treated with hysterectomy — the surgical removal of the uterus. Along with the uterus, the surgeon may also remove the ovaries, fallopian tubes, and selected lymph nodes.

Abnormal Uterine Bleeding

Abnormal uterine bleeding can adversely affect a woman's well-being and quality of life. Sometimes the abnormal bleeding is a warning sign for uterine cancer or pre-cancer, but this condition can also occur with uterine fibroids, polyps, abnormal pregnancy, and certain types of infcctions. Conservative (non-surgical) medical therapy is the first line of treatment for many of these non-cancerous conditions, but when non-invasive methods fail, a hysterectomy may be a viable option.

Pelvic Organ Prolapse

Pelvic organ prolapse is sometimes referred to as a "dropped bladder," cystocele, rectocele, enterocele, or proccidentia. This occurs because the tissues that hold the vagina and uterus in place have become disrupted, usually related to childbirth followed by aging. Because of this, the vagina turns "inside out", and shows up as tissues appearing to "fall out" of the vagina. This problem is a mechanical one, and is usually treated by resuspending the vagina, often with removal of part, or all, of the uterus that amounts to a total or supracervical hysterectomy.

Pelvic Pain – Endometriosis and Adenomyosis

Pelvic pain related to an enlarged or painful uterus, can sometimes be caused by endometriosis or another condition called adenomyosis. Endometriosis and adenomyosis are similar conditions in which the tissues (cells) that normally line the uterus (the endometrium), inhabit organs and areas well away from the uterine lining. If the endometrial tissue covers the ovaries, tubes, bladder, or other pelvic structures, this is called endometriosis. If the endometrial tissue burrows into the uterine muscle, this is called adenomyosis. Both conditions can sometimes result in debilitating pelvic pain, usually worse around the time of menstrual periods. These conditions are treated initially with medications, but if medication therapy fails, hysterectomy may be an option for treatment.

Fibroids

Fibroids are growths of non-cancerous cells that sometimes grow into the muscle of the uterus. They can sometimes become quite large, and can cause pain, abnormal bleeding, as well as low back pain, pressure and bladder problems. When fibroids cause severe symptoms, medical and other non-invasive therapies are used to try to improve the symptoms. When these therapies fail, surgical options include removal of the fibroids (myomectomy) or removal of the uterus (hysterectomy). The choice of therapy depends on the needs of the patient and the capabilities of the surgeon.

6

Extent of a Hysterectomy

IF A HYSTERECTOMY IS RECOMMENDED, several options are available, depending on patient needs and the clinical situation. Hysterectomy can be performed in three basic ways: total hysterectomy, subtotal (or supracervical) hysterectomy, and radical hysterectomy.

Each technique carries its own benefits and drawbacks. Depending on the type of female issue involved, your surgeon may recommend removal of the ovaries and tubes at the time of hysterectomy. Every woman facing hysterectomy needs to understand the anatomy or arrangement of the pelvic organs, so that she can make an informed decision regarding the extent of tissue removal needed to correct the problem.

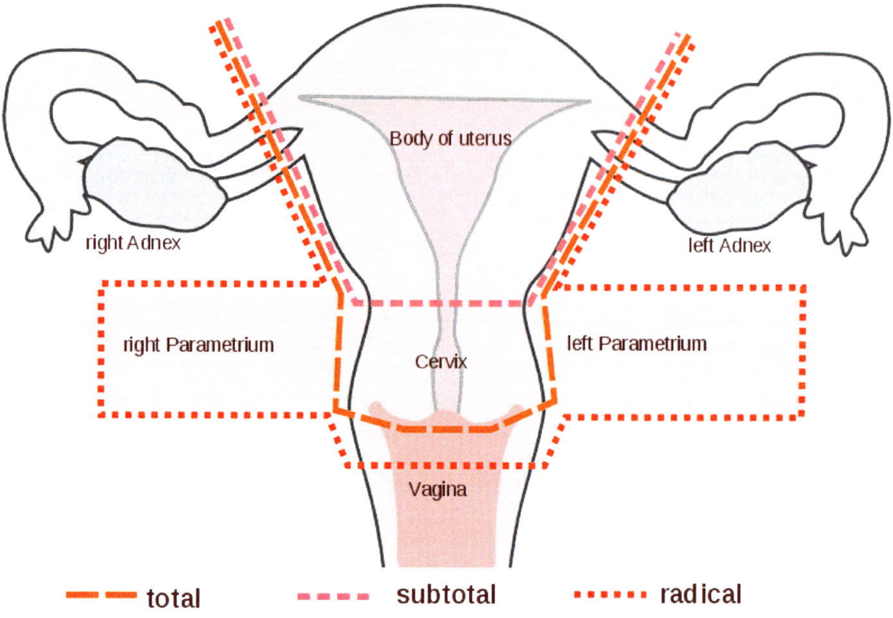

This Illustrates the Three Types of Hysterectomies

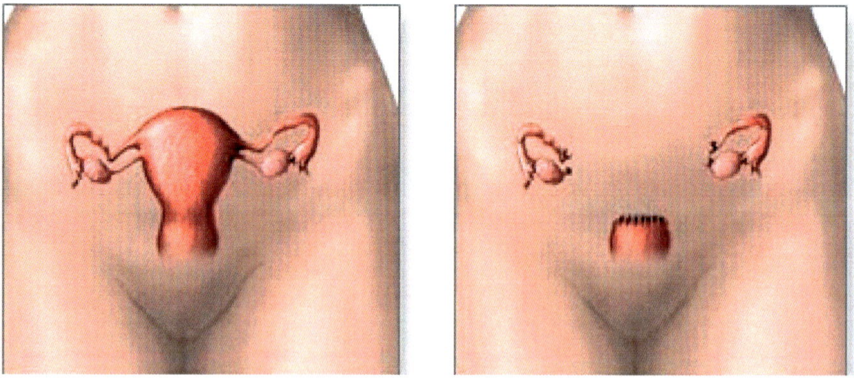

The Uterus Surgically Removed during a Hysterectomy

A hysterectomy involves partial or complete removal of a woman's uterus or womb. The uterus has two parts, the fundus (top part), and the cervix (bottom part). The upper end of the cervix is connected to the uterus, and this connection is called the isthmus. The lower end of the cervix connects directly to the vagina. To the right and left of the upper part of the uterus, the fallopian tubes and the ovaries are located. There is usually a fallopian tube and an ovary on each side. The ovaries produce eggs and hormones, which regulate the menstrual cycle and other important functions. The fallopian tubes carry eggs from the ovaries to the uterus. As a point of reference, these organs are located in a woman's lower abdomen, as shown in the illustration.

Total Hysterectomy

For the total hysterectomy, the uterus along with the cervix is removed. This can be performed as an open, vaginal or laparoscopic/robotic procedure. The supracervical (subtotal) hysterectomy involves separating (cutting) the uterus from the cervix, and removing the uterus. The cervix is the lower end of the uterus that joins the vagina. This procedure can be done as an open or laparoscopic/robotic procedure. With a supracervical hysterectomy, because the cervix is left in place, some women may have monthly spotting from the cells that line the inside of the cervix.

Radical Hysterectomy

The radical hysterectomy involves removal of the uterus, cervix, and upper vagina, along with the tissues on either side that support the uterus and cervix (also called the parametrium). This procedure is normally performed by the open, laparoscopic, or robotic method.

Sometimes the surgeon may recommend removal of the ovaries and fallopian tubes, depending on the clinical situation, usually after an extensive discussion with the woman. Unless there is a serious problem with the ovaries, these are not usually removed at the time of hysterectomy in pre-menopausal women.

Following total or radical hysterectomy, a woman will no longer have periods.

Robotic Versus Laparoscopic Hysterectomy Surgery

While "straight stick" laparoscopy offers a minimally invasive approach in the hands of a skilled surgeon, it limits the surgeon's ability to address complex uterine pathology such as large fibroids, large uteruses, complex suturing (stitching) and the complex dissection required in cancer surgery. With the advanced 3D vision system, flexible instruments, and decreased surgeon discomfort, the robotic system allows the surgeon to see inside the abdomen and perform complex, advanced surgical operations in the confined space.

By overcoming the limitations of both traditional open, vaginal, and laparoscopic surgery, robotic surgery is redefining gynecologic surgery for women.

Most gynecologic surgeons agree that when a hysterectomy is needed, the best approach for the woman is a minimally invasive approach when compared to open surgery. Minimally invasive approaches include the laparoscopic and robotic approaches. Despite several decades of exposure to laparoscopic surgery, as mentioned earlier, today, open hysterectomy is still the method used to perform the majority of hysterectomies in the United States. Many believe that this is because of the difficulty in gaining the kind of surgical exposure required to deal with the more complex uterine pathology.

There is also the steep curve associated with learning the laparoscopic technique, and the inherent physical strains on the laparoscopic surgeon. In fact, studies suggest that the experienced, high volume laparoscopic surgeon is much more likely to suffer from musculoskeletal disorders related to surgical posture, compared to the less-experienced laparoscopist.

Reference: Patients Benefit While Surgeons Suffer: An Impending Epidemic □Adrian Park, Gyusung Lee, F. Jacob Seagull, Nora Meenaghan, David Dexter □Journal of the American College of Surgeons - March 2010 (Vol. 210, Issue 3, Pages 306-313, DOI: 10.1016/j.jamcollsurg.2009.10.017)

Data suggests that there are advantages in using the robotic surgical technique, over "straight stick" laparoscopy, both for the surgeon's well-being, and for the patient.

The following table displays patient outcomes for hysterectomy for benign gynecologic conditions. As you can see, *da Vinci* Hysterectomy shows measurable advantages as compared to both traditional open surgery performed through a large abdominal incision and conventional minimally invasive laparoscopic surgery (referred to as laparoscopy).

Outcome Comparison: *da Vinci®* vs. Laparoscopy vs. Open Surgery

Comparative Data	*da Vinci*[12] (n = 100)	Laparoscopy[12] (n = 100)	Open[12] (n = 5,875)
Operative times (minutes)	78.7*	92.4	86.1
Estimated blood loss (ml)	61.1	113.0	305.1
% of patients requiring open surgery**	4%	20%	Not applicable
Complications %	2%	2%	17.2%
Average length of hospital stay (days)	1.1	1.6	6.0

**Last 25 procedures*
***The percent of patients who required open abdominal surgery whose condition was not amenable to a minimally invasive approach using da Vinci (4%) or laparoscopy (20%).*

What does it mean?

- *da Vinci* hysterectomy can reduce hospital stay, minimize blood loss, and reduce the risk of surgical complications compared to open abdominal surgery for benign gynecologic conditions.
- Only four percent of *da Vinci* hysterectomy patients required conversion to open surgery, but with laparoscopy, twenty per-

cent (five times as many) required conversion to open surgery. This data demonstrates that *da Vinci* surgery will enable gynecologists to treat even complex or more advanced conditions using minimally invasive techniques.

- Unlike conventional laparoscopy, *da Vinci* allows gynecologists to treat patients with more advanced benign pathology, such as an enlarged uterus (e.g., due to fibroids or adenomyosis) and pelvic adhesive disease (e.g., due to endometriosis or prior pelvic surgeries). This, in turn, will allow gynecologists to extend the benefits of minimally invasive surgery to more patient types.
- Ultimately, Robotic Surgery will allow gynecologists to perform fewer open abdominal surgeries for hysterectomy.

Part Three

The Robotic Surgical Procedures

7

The Robotic Hysterectomy Procedure

A HYSTERECTOMY (ablation; cutting out; extirpation; excision) is the removal of the uterus. This is surgery performed for several conditions, detailed earlier, in and surrounding the uterus. It is one of the most commonly performed procedures in the country.

The surgical technique of hysterectomy involves a three-step process. First, the blood vessels feeding the uterus are tied off and cut. Second, the organs that lie close the uterus (bladder, bowels, ovaries) are gently moved out of the way. Third, the tissues that hold the uterus in place (the supports or pedicles), are tied off and cut. In this way, the uterus is carefully removed from the pelvis in a way that seeks to minimize blood loss and damage to nearby organs and needed tissues.

The blood supply to the uterus comes, in part, from the ovarian blood supply (ovarian artery and vein), and in part from the blood vessels that come directly to the uterus (the uterine artery and vein). In most women, the ovarian blood supply enters the uterus at the upper portion, and the uterine artery and vein enters the uterus near the junction of the uterus and cervix. The uterus is held in place by several tissue links, called ligaments. These include the round ligament and the utero-ovarian ligament which attach near the top of the uterus, and cardinal ligament, which attaches near the middle of the uterus. The cardinal ligament carries the uterine artery and vein. Another ligament, called the broad ligament, covers the entire uterus like a drape, and helps to hold it in place. Down at the level of the cervix, the uterus is attached to the vagina, such that the opening of the cervix faces down into the canal, or opening in the vagina.

During the robotic hysterectomy, the wristed instruments are used to coagulate (burn), and then cut the round ligaments. The coagulation is used to prevent bleeding when the ligament is cut. The same thing is done to the utero-ovarian ligaments (which contain blood supply from the ovaries), followed by the uterine artery and veins and the broad ligament. The bladder is then gently dissected (pushed) off of the lower part of the uterus and cervix, which then exposes the place where the cervix and vagina meet.

For the total hysterectomy, the cervix is then cut away from the vagina at the place where they meet, again using the wristed robotic instruments. The uterus and cervix can then be pulled through the vagina by the assistant. The cut edges of the vagina are then stitched closed using the robotic instruments. The robot arms and ports are then removed, and the skin incisions are closed, either with sutures (stitches), or special skin glue.

For a supracervical hysterectomy, the robotic scissors are used to cut the uterus at the junction with the cervix, separating the upper part of the uterus (the fundus) from the cervix. The uterus is then morcellated (cut into small pieces) and the small pieces are removed through the port controlled by the assistant. The cut edge of the cervix is then either closed over with stitches, or cauterized (burned) with an electrical device to prevent bleeding. The lining of the cervix is also cauterized to remove the glandular cells that can sometimes cause irregular vaginal bleeding.

The radical hysterectomy resembles the total hysterectomy, except that the connecting pedicles (supporting tissues) are tied off and cut further away from the uterus itself, to try and get any cancer cells that may have grown into the supporting tissues and ligaments. The upper part of the vagina is also removed during a radical hysterectomy. Because of the wider extent of the tissue removal, the radical hysterectomy carries an increased risk of affecting the bladder's ability to empty itself after the surgery. However, some surgeons report a lower risk of bladder problems after robotic radical hysterectomy, compared to open or laparoscopic radical hysterectomy.

Extent of a Hysterectomy

A surgeon may choose to remove all, or only part, of the uterus. It is important for patients and health care providers to communicate effectively and to have clarity regarding whether the cervix and/or tubes and ovaries are to be removed:

- In a supracervical or subtotal hysterectomy, a surgeon removes only the upper part of the uterus, keeping the cervix in place.
- A total hysterectomy removes the whole uterus and cervix.
- In a radical hysterectomy, a surgeon removes the whole uterus, tissue on the sides of the uterus, the cervix, and the top part of the vagina. Radical hysterectomy is generally performed when cervical cancer is present.

Removal of an ovary is called an oopherectomy, and removal of a fallopian tube is called a salpingectomy. Removal of the tube and ovary often are done together, and this is called a salpingo-oopherectomy. Unilateral refers to one side, and bilateral refers to both sides. A left (or right) unilateral salpingo-oopherectomy means that the tube and ovary on the left (or right) side were removed. A bilateral salpingo-oopherectomy means that the tubes and ovaries on both sides were removed.

8

Preparing For Robotic Surgery

BEFORE YOU CAN UNDERGO surgery, including robotic surgery, there are many details that need to be taken care of in advance. Your surgeon will need to be sure that you are healthy enough to undergo surgery safely. You will need to have all of your medications evaluated to see which ones can be safely taken up to the time of surgery, and which ones need to be stopped in advance of surgery. In the two days leading up to your surgery, many surgeons will ask you to prepare your bowels for surgery. You will also need to stop eating and drinking on the night before surgery. All of this information will be explained verbally to you, and also given to you in the form of a written sheet of instructions.

Ensuring That You Are Healthy for Surgery

The hysterectomy is usually considered to be an elective procedure, which means that it is not an emergency. Before any elective surgery, your surgeon will want to know that your body is strong enough to handle the stress. If you are generally healthy, with no other medical problems, your surgeon will require you to have a simple blood test to show that your blood levels are appropriate. This test is called a Complete Blood Count (CBC), and it tells your surgeon that your blood will carry enough oxygen to keep your heart functioning during and after surgery, and to help your tissues heal. The CBC will also report on your blood clotting ability, and let the surgeon know that you do not have any infections that might make the surgery unsafe for you. If you are still having periods, your doctor will also ask for a urine pregnancy test to make sure that you are not pregnant at the time of surgery.

If you are over 65, your doctor may choose to get a chest X-ray to make sure that your lungs are clear, and also an EKG to make sure that your heart is working well. If you have high blood pressure, or are taking medications for other medical problems, your doctor may want to get additional blood tests to study your liver and kidney function.

If you have any problems with your heart, lungs, liver, or kidneys, your surgeon may request surgical clearance from a specialist such as a cardiologist, pulmonologist, or liver or kidney specialist. In this case, the specialist will examine you thoroughly, and perform special tests if needed, to make sure that you will remain safe during your surgery. Once your specialist is satisfied that your surgery can proceed safely, they will communicate their findings in a letter to your surgeon.

If you have diabetes, your surgeon will make a special effort to make sure your blood sugar is well controlled before, during, and in the days and weeks after your surgery. Keeping your blood sugar under control is important because this can affect how well your tissues heal after surgery.

Medical and Surgical History Review

It is very important that you tell your surgeon about any medical conditions with which you have been diagnosed, or for which you have been, or are being treated. Even if you had a medical condition in the past, that is no longer active, you need to tell your surgeon. The stress of surgery can sometimes reactivate these conditions, potentially with life threatening consequences. Asthma, diabetes, heart attacks, abnormal heart rhythms, heart murmurs, COPD, surgeries (including cosmetic surgeries), and reactions to anesthesia are all conditions that your surgeon needs to know about in order to keep you safe during surgery. Your surgeon will also need to know what medications you are taking, and also what, if any, allergies you have to medications.

Medication Review

Many medications are safe to take up to the day before surgery. Other medications can affect your blood's clotting function, and need to be stopped or changed well in advance of your surgery. Blood thinners make it harder for your blood to clot, and can lead to too much bleeding at the time of surgery. Some blood thinners like Coumadin™ (warfarin) are long acting, and need to be stopped about seven days prior to surgery. If you need to have your blood thinned, your surgeon will switch you over to a short acting blood thinner like Heparin or Lovenox ™, which you can take up to the day before surgery. With these short acting medications, your blood thinning will wear off over a twenty-four hour period, allowing your surgery to take place safely. Once your surgery is completed, your surgeon will restart your long acting blood thinner.

If you take a daily anti-platelet agent, like aspirin or Plavix™, to help prevent blood clots in your heart or brain arteries, your surgeon may safely stop the aspirin or Plavix seven to ten days before your surgery. (However, if you have stents in the blood vessels of your heart you cannot stop the Plavix or aspirin.) Only your surgeon can decide if your Plavix or aspirin need to be stopped prior to surgery. This decision depends heavily on your individual medical condition, so be sure to ask your surgeon before stopping any medication.

It is very important that you tell your surgeon about every single medication that you are taking. This includes over-the-counter medications like ibuprofen (Motrin), and also herbal remedies, as these can affect your body functions during and after surgery.

Only your surgeon and your anesthesiologist can decide which medications need to be stopped prior to surgery.

Diet Pills

It is very important to realize that diet medications – pills, injections and other preparations — can affect your body's response to anesthetic agents and medications designed to control your body functions during and after surgery. Diet medications can be harmful to you around the time of surgery. These medications need to be stopped two weeks prior to your surgery. You need to tell your surgeon about any dieting activities that you are engaged in, well in advance of your surgery.

Your Preoperative Visit

Your preoperative visit involves sitting down with your surgeon to go over the type of surgery planned, and the reasons for the surgery. This is the time to ask any questions you have regarding your surgery. Your surgeon will be ready to answer your questions and give you lots of information about what to expect during your surgery and afterwards, including your recovery, and the period after that. Your surgeon will discuss how your body will change, and what to expect after you have recovered from surgery.

Most surgeons will require you to meet with the anesthesiologist and hospital team several days before your surgery. This is called the preoperative (pre-op) visit. In this visit, your anesthesiologist will go over your medical history, and examine you to make sure that it is safe to put you under anesthesia. Your anesthesiologist will review any clearance letters from your cardiologist or other specialist, to make sure that your surgery can be done safely. If not already done, your blood tests will also be drawn on this visit. Often, you will be asked to give your written consent for your surgery during your pre-op visit. Make sure you understand the planned surgery, including the reason, and what to expect after surgery. The preoperative visit is a good time to make sure that you understand what the surgery will do, the reasons for doing the surgery, what to expect after surgery, and the alternatives to surgery. Do not be afraid to ask any questions that you may have related to your surgery.

Just Before Your Surgery

Many surgeons will ask that you take a medication to clean your bowels out prior to your robotic surgery. If your bowels are cleaned out, it makes it easier for your surgeon to perform your surgery robotically. Some surgeons will ask you to do a two-day bowel prep, and others use a one-day prep. The prep consists of a liquid like magnesium citrate, or GoLYTELY™.

For the two-day bowel prep, you would consume a liquid diet for two days prior to surgery. At around 4:00 p.m. on the day before surgery, you would drink either two bottles of magnesium citrate, or a bottle of GoLYTELY, which will cause you to have loose, watery stool for several hours. You should not plan any activities outside the home once you drink the bowel prep medications, because you will need to go to the bathroom frequently..

Most surgeons demand that you have nothing to eat or drink after midnight on the night before your surgery. This is important because your stomach needs to be completely empty when you go under anesthesia. If your stomach is not completely empty, stomach acids can travel to your lungs when you are put under anesthesia, potentially causing serious, life threatening harm to your lungs. If you need to take a medication on the morning of surgery, your surgeon will usually let you take it with a small sip of pure water. It is important to know that most surgeons will cancel your surgery if you have takien anything by mouth after midnight on the day before your surgery.

The Day of Surgery

On the day of surgery, you will be asked to arrive two hours before the time that your surgery is scheduled. You will be brought to the preoperative area, where you will be checked into the hospital and interviewed by a nurse. The nurse will verify your identity, your surgeon, and the procedure that you are having. She will also review your medical history, including your medications, and allergies. If you have brought any valuables with you, these can be given to someone who came with you for safekeeping. Sometimes, your valuables will be placed with hospital security until after your surgery is over and you have recovered well enough to take charge of them.

Once you have been interviewed by the nurse, you will be asked to put on a hospital gown, and an IV will be placed into one of the veins in your arm, in order to give you fluids. At this time, your anesthesiology team will come to visit with you, and briefly explain the process of going under anesthesia. Your surgeon will also come to see you, confirm that all of your questions have been answered, and ensure that your informed consent form reflects the surgery that is planned. Once these things are completed, you will be ready to be moved into the operating room for your surgery.

Additional Preparation Suggestions

- **Be informed** - find out as much as you can from the medical team about your operation. Do not be afraid to ask questions; they are used to this and should gladly explain everything and respond to any queries you may have.
- **Get help** - if you live alone, or the other household members are not able to assist you, arrange for a friend or relative to come and help you at home for the first week or two after the operation.
- **Household Items** - organize your home for when you return. Place all your most-used objects in an easy-to-access place,

such as your TV remote, radio, telephone, medications, tissues, address book, eyeglasses, pens, paper, etc.

- **Organize your provisions** - make sure you have plenty of canned, frozen, and easy-to-prepare foods for your return. If somebody is going to help look after you, check this with them.
- **Hygiene** - have a shower and put clean clothes on before you leave the house to come to the hospital. This helps prevent bringing unwanted bacteria into the hospital.
- **Nails** - make sure your finger and toenails are clipped. During your operation you will be under general anesthetic; you will be moved around on a trolley, unable to prevent a toe or finger from sticking out of the side.
- **Dietary requirements** - if you are vegetarian, vegan, or have any special dietary requirements, it is important that you let the hospital know about this well in advance. When you get to the hospital, check to be sure that they have not forgotten.

Medication

Please read and follow your surgeon's medication instructions carefully

- Bring all medications in their labeled containers with you on the day of your preoperative visit and surgery. If you are taking aspirin, Motrin, Coumadin, herbal remedies (e.g., St. John's Wort, garlic, Vitamin E) or other medications, ask your surgeon if you need to stop these before your surgery. Be sure to do this at least two weeks prior to your planned surgery date.

Bowel Management

- Follow your surgeon's instructions regarding what to eat in the 2 days prior to surgery.
- Follow your surgeon's instructions for bowel prep.

- DO NOT eat or drink anything after MIDNIGHT on the night before surgery, including water, juice, coffee, chewing gum or candy.

Other Preparations:

- Leave jewelry and other valuables at home. If you wear contact lenses, glasses, or false teeth, you must bring your case to store them in during surgery.

Please bring:

- Insurance card/authorization number/copayment.
- Any other papers your physician has given you.
- List of current medicines (with dosages) and any medicine allergies.
- Copies of EKG and/or chest X-ray done in the past year.
- Completed health questionnaire.

In Addition

- Notify your physician of any changes in your health such as a cold, fever, flu or other illnesses.
- Arrange for a ride home. Patients receiving any type of anesthesia or sedation are not allowed to drive home. We recommend, for your safety, that you have a responsible adult stay with you for twenty-four hours after surgery.
- No smoking within twenty-four hours of surgery.
- No food, water, hard candy, chewing gum or tobacco after the specified time. Brushing teeth is permitted the morning of surgery. Rinse and spit; do not swallow water.
- Do not wear make-up or jewelry.
- Remove nail polish.
- Please bring your hearing aids to the hospital.

- Please bring your inhaler to the hospital, if you use one for asthma or other reasons.
- If you wear glasses or contact lenses, bring them (and your case and contact solution).
- If your doctor wants you to use crutches after surgery, please bring them on the day of your operation.

Arrival Time

Arrive at the hospital one to two hours prior to your scheduled surgery. Wear loose, comfortable clothing. You will be asked to change into a hospital gown; the gown ties in the back. You will be given a sheet or blanket to cover yourself. A nurse will verify your diagnosis, surgery, surgical site, and that your signature is on the necessary documents. Complete the informed consent, and certify that you have followed instructions on eating and drinking restrictions. Your allergies will be verified. This includes allergies to medicines and latex. A brief physical assessment will be completed. Notify your nurse if your health has changed since your pre-admit visit or telephone appointment.

9

Your Robotic-Assisted Surgery

WHEN YOU ARRIVE AT THE HOSPITAL, YOU CAN expect to go through a checklist of pre-surgery instructions. On the day before surgery, you will have had a bowel preparation that involves drinking a liquid which causes mechanical bowel cleansing. This procedure reduces bowel distention, and reduces the natural movements of your bowels, making it easier to keep the bowels out of the way during the surgical procedure. Bowel cleansing may also reduce the potential for infection that could occur in the unlikely event of bowel injury during surgery.

In the Pre-op Area

After you check in for surgery, you will be asked to change into a hospital gown. For women of reproductive age, you will be asked to provide a urine sample for a urine pregnancy test. Once the urine pregnancy test is negative, your nurse or anesthesiologist will place an intravenous (IV) line in one of the veins in your arm, and will begin running fluids through the IV. The fluids are designed to keep you from becoming dehydrated. Your nurse will also place special stockings on your legs, as well as special inflatable leg covers called sequential compression devices (SCD). The stockings and SCDs help reduce the risk of developing blood clots during, and after, surgery.

Your nurse will then review the planned procedure with you, to confirm that you understand the surgery that is planned and the reason for the surgery. Your surgeon will also visit you in the PREOP area to review the planned procedure and answer any questions you may have. Once your surgical consent is verified, and your questions are answered, you will be ready for surgery. At this time, your anesthesiologist may choose to run a sedative medication through your IV to help you relax. Many surgeons will request that you receive an antibiotic in your IV to help reduce the risk of infection related to surgery.

In the Operating Room (OR)

At this time, you will be taken into the operating room, and placed on the surgical table, facing the ceiling. You will be asked to hold a special breathing mask over your nose and mouth, which will supply you with oxygen. Your anesthesiologist will then begin to place the anesthetic medication into your IV, and you will slowly drift off to sleep. Once you are asleep, you will be given medication so that you cannot feel any pain. You will also be given a muscle-relaxing medication, and a breathing tube will be placed into your windpipe (trachea), so that you can be given oxygen and anesthetic gas. Most importantly, the breathing tube will be attached to a special machine that will inflate your lungs to provide oxygen, and deflate them to remove carbon dioxide. In this way, the machine breathes for you during the surgery while you are under anesthetic. The breathing tube is secured in your windpipe using a special sticky tape to tape it to your mouth.

Once you are under anesthesia, and the tube is secured, the OR team will place you in the correct position for your surgery to begin. This usually involves placing your feet in special boots called stirrups, which allow your surgeon to have access to the vaginal area so that your uterus can be manipulated as needed during surgery. At this time, a special antibiotic liquid will be used to paint your abdomen, pubic, and vaginal area to help prevent infection of the surgical incisions. Once this liquid dries, your body will be covered with a sterile surgical drape, which will expose only the area that was painted. This will be the area that the surgeon will place the special incisions for the robotic instruments. A catheter will be placed in your bladder to drain your urine throughout the surgical procedure.

Surgery may require a surgeon, an assistant surgeon, an anesthesiologist, and one or two nurses. Most robotic surgeries have one surgeon at the console and the assistant surgeon next to the patient guiding the robotic arms, removing tissues, and passing sutures to the robotic instruments.

The surgeon makes five to six 1-centimeter skin incisions in the lower abdomen. The EndoWrist instruments and high definition camera are introduced in the body through these laparoscopic ports.

The first incision is usually at, or above, the belly button. A needle is passed through this incision, and is used to pass carbon dioxide gas into the abdomen to inflate it, allowing the surgeon to clearly see the tissues and organs of interest. Once the abdomen is inflated, the needle is removed and a larger one-half to one-centimeter cylinder (trochar) is passed through the needle hole. The robotic camera is then passed through this trochar, and is used to see inside the abdomen. At this time, you will be repositioned so that your head is placed much lower than your abdomen, such that the bowels fall away from the pelvis towards your head. This allows your surgeon to see your uterus, tubes, and ovaries easily, and in fine detail. Using this camera as a guide, your surgeon will place three to four more incisions and trochars into your abdomen, so that the robotic instruments can be inserted later. The bed will then be tilted so that your head is lower than your pelvis. This moves your bowels out of the way so you're your pelvic organs can be clearly seen.

Once these trochars are placed, and the bed has been tilted backwards, the *da Vinci* robot is then brought into position, close to the patient, and the robot arms are connected to the trochars. Once the robot arms are connected, the EndoWrist instruments are placed through the trochar ports, and your surgery can begin. The high-definition 3D camera, and three other instruments, will be under the direct control of your surgeon during the surgical procedure.

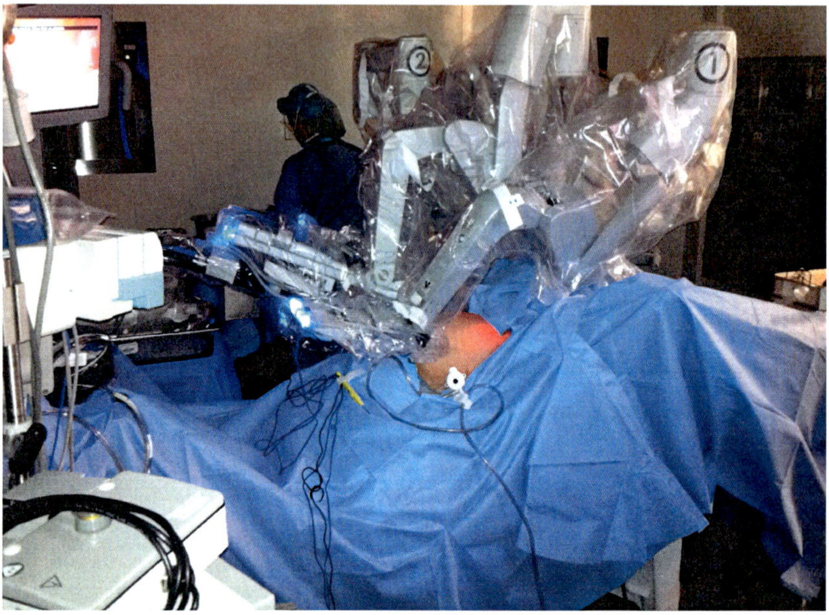

Patient on table prepared for robotic surgery

Once all the instruments, and the surgical assistant, are prepared, the surgeon will move to the console that is at a distance from the patient on the operating table. The surgeon will seat himself/herself on the chair that is part of the console. With the fixed binoculars, the surgeon will check the view being transmitted by the camera inside the abdomen. The surgical assistant will check the scene on the monitor on a side cart next to the patient.

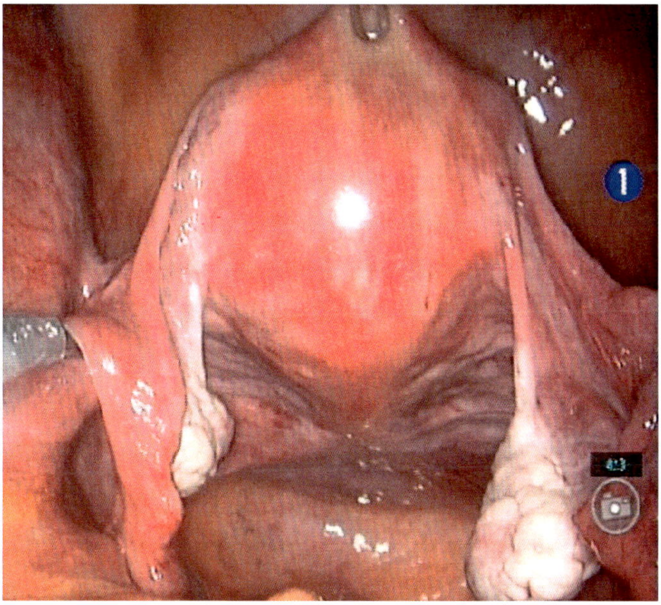

Image of the uterus-pink, ovaries, white, and tubes-pink as seen on the monitor. *©2010 Lennox Hoyte MD.*

The surgeon puts his/her head in the viewing camera. At the surgeon's disposal are three robotic arms and a 3D camera that can move around inside the body. Rather than programming the robot to make surgical maneuvers, the surgeon manually dictates the robot's every move.

Robotic arms clutch the surgical instruments inside the patient's body. A computer transmits the surgeon's movements to the robot instruments, and they carry out the surgeon's orders immediately. It's an exact duplication; there's no delay, It's happening at exactly the same time. The surgeon's hand movements correspond directly to the movements of the robotic instruments during the entire procedure.

During the robotic surgery, various instruments may be inserted into the trochar ports to retract, cut, suture and staple the tissues as directed by the surgeron (this is all done while the patient is asleep). Unlike conventional laparoscopic surgery, the surgeon does not touch these surgical instruments directly.

Sitting at the control console a few feet from the operating table, the surgeon looks into a viewfinder. The camera inside the patient allows the surgeon to explore the narrow structures of the body in three dimensions. The images show the surgical site and the two or three surgical instruments connected to the robotic arms. The surgeon uses joystick-like controls located underneath the screen to manipulate the surgical instruments.

Each time the surgeon moves one of the joysticks, a computer sends an electronic signal to one of the instruments, which moves in sync with the movements of the surgeon's hands. In this way, the surgeon uses the robot to perform complete surgical procedures without the need for large incisions.

Because of the magnification, 3D visualization, and wristed instruments, the surgeon can more easily identify, manipulate, and cut tissues to disconnect the uterus from the vagina, supports, and blood vessels, while minimizing damage to vital nearby structures.

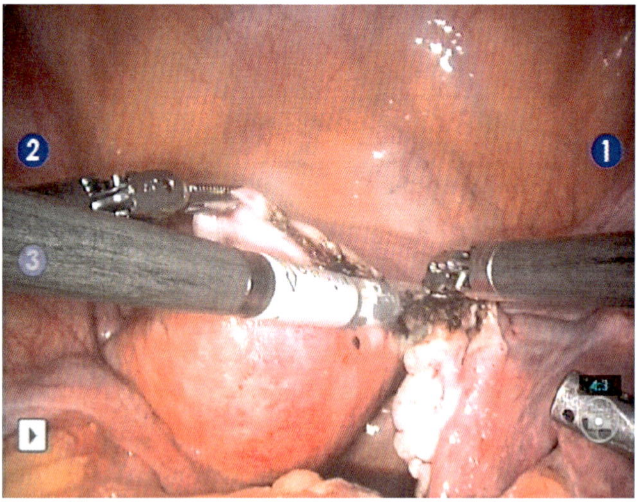

The right sided uterine pedicles disconnected.

Once the uterus is disconnected from its supports and blood supply, the detached uterus will be pulled out through the vagina by the assistant. The surgeon can then close the cut edges of the vagina with the robotic instruments using sutures passed in by the assistant. In the case of a supracervical hysterectomy, the uterus is cut up and removed in pieces through the assistant port.

Once this is completed, the surgeon will survey the surgical area to ensure that the tissues are hemostatic (not bleeding). Once this is verified, it will be time to remove the instruments, disconnect the robot, remove the air from the abdomen, remove the trocar ports, and close the incisions with fine sutures. These sutures usually dissolve after a few weeks. Sometimes, surgical glue will be used to close the incisions instead of sutures. Most robotic hysterectomies will be completed in one to two hours. Once the robot is removed, the patient's body is returned to a normal horizontal position.

When suturing is completed, the anesthesia will be reversed, and the breathing tube will be removed when the patient is sufficiently alert to breathe on her own. After the tube is removed, the patient is taken to the recovery room.

10

Safe Robotic Surgery

WHEN CONSIDERING SURGICAL TREATMENT options, many patients have concerns about safety. In particular, patients question whether *da Vinci* surgery is as safe as traditional methods. It has been proven safe. In fact, the *da Vinci* Robotic Surgical System has been used successfully in tens of thousands of minimally invasive procedures worldwide. Multiple, redundant safety features make *da Vinci* potentially as safe as traditional methods, if not more so. Still, it is important to realize that surgery and anesthesia carry real risks as well as benefits. Both need to be considered in detail before a woman decides to proceed with surgery. Make sure your surgeon is aware of every medical condition that you have or had in the past, even if you are not being treated for it currently.

Surgeon-Controlled Robotic System

First and foremost, the *da Vinci* System cannot be programmed, nor can it make decisions on its own. Instead, the *da Vinci* System requires that every surgical maneuver be performed with direct input from the surgeon. The surgeon performs the surgery — not the robot.

The arms of the robot are extremely nimble and are manipulated by the surgeon using joystick-like controls. The robot also has a camera that gives the surgeon a magnified 3D view. Very small blood vessels and nerves can be seen clearly and can be spared, as needed.

The hand movements of the surgeon are duplicated in the patient by the robot, but on a much smaller scale. The robotic instruments are used to cut away tissue, cauterize blood vessels, and place sutures, using needles held by pincer-like "needle drivers." The robot's wrist can turn nearly 360 degrees, allowing great flexibility. The robot also eliminates any tremors in a surgeon's hands, and, for delicate work, "motion scaling" software reduces a surgeon's actual hand movements to much smaller, finer, instrument movements. Robot-assisted surgery allows the surgeon greater dexterity and control over very fine movements than traditional laparoscopy.

Robotic surgery's instruments with distal ends, or tips, are unique. They mimic the intricate movements of the human hand, while at the same time providing the surgeon with a high-definition, three-dimensional view of the operative field.

One doctor mentioned, "The surgeon performing surgery with instrumentation and technology is not very different from having your actual arms and hands working the patient's abdominal cavity. Since the pelvis is a very narrow place with uterus, bladder, bowel and structures that can easily be injured, precision and the ability to articulate as well as visualize — is critically important."

Shared-control robotic systems permit two surgeons to work together during surgery, but the surgeons do most of the work. Unlike automatic robotic systems that perform other tasks without manual intervention, the surgeons must operate the surgical instruments themselves. The robotic system provides stability and mechanical support of the instruments.

The robot handles the laparoscope and instruments, while the surgeon controls the actions of the instruments from the console. Glove-like devices on the surgeon's hands respond to finger movements and twists of the hands and wrists. Most surgeons agree that for complex hysterectomies, robot-assisted surgery is more effective and less invasive.

Unlikely System Failure

During the course of an operation, the *da Vinci* Surgical System will perform millions of safety self-checks. The system is designed to be fail-safe, which means that in the event of power interruption or a safety-check failure, the system shuts down safely, allowing the surgeon to remain in control of the procedure.

If, for any reason, the surgeon senses there is a malfunction, or if the surgeon senses that it is not safe to continue, the robotic system will be withdrawn and the surgery will proceed either with the laparoscopic method or traditional open surgery. This requires that the surgeon be highly skilled at laparoscopy, as well as open surgical technique, in the unlikely event that the surgical approach needs to be converted to one or the other. The surgeon must master open and/or laparoscopic gynecologic surgery before undergoing the multiple stages of special training to gain mastery of the robotic surgical system.

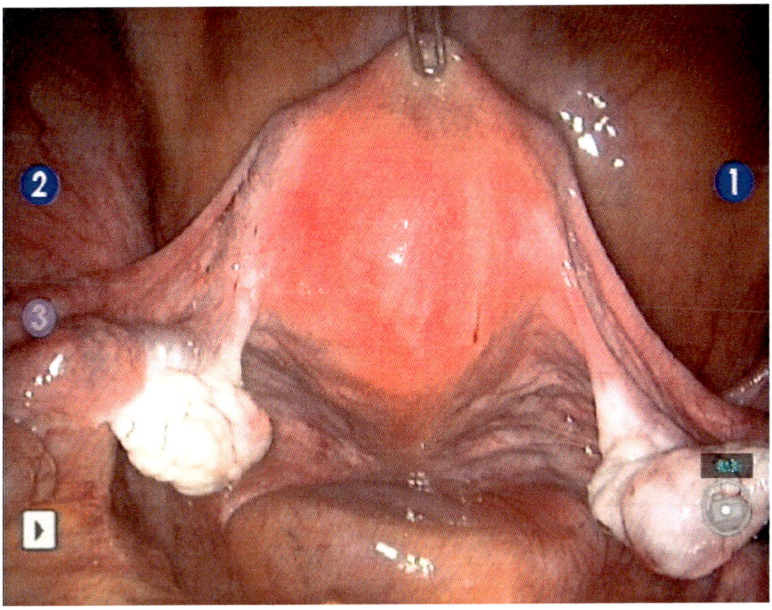

The Surgeon's View relayed by the camera during Surgery.

The highly precise movements of the robotic arms allow for cleaner removal of cancerous tissues. Such precision also produces a more targeted approach which reduces damage to healthy tissue during the operation. The design of the robotic operating arms allows for the entire procedure to be conducted without having to leverage operating tools against the walls of the incision. This can decrease postoperative pain at the site of the incisions.

In contrast to earlier laparoscopic tools, which had limited range of motion, the *da Vinci* surgical instruments exceed the movement capabilities of the human hand with the added bonus of mechanical precision. The robotic arms can rotate a full 360 degrees. The *da Vinci* interface translates each movement of the surgeon's hands on the controls into precise movements of these micro-instruments. The system is so sophisticated that it can distinguish between hand tremors and intentional hand movements.

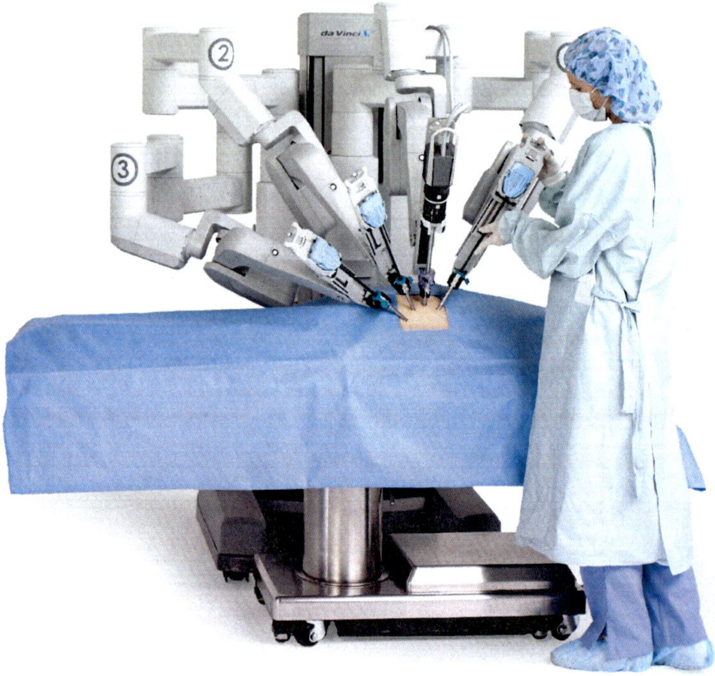

Nurse at da Vinci Patient Cart

Once the surgery is complete, the surgeons remove the rods from the patient's body and close the incisions.

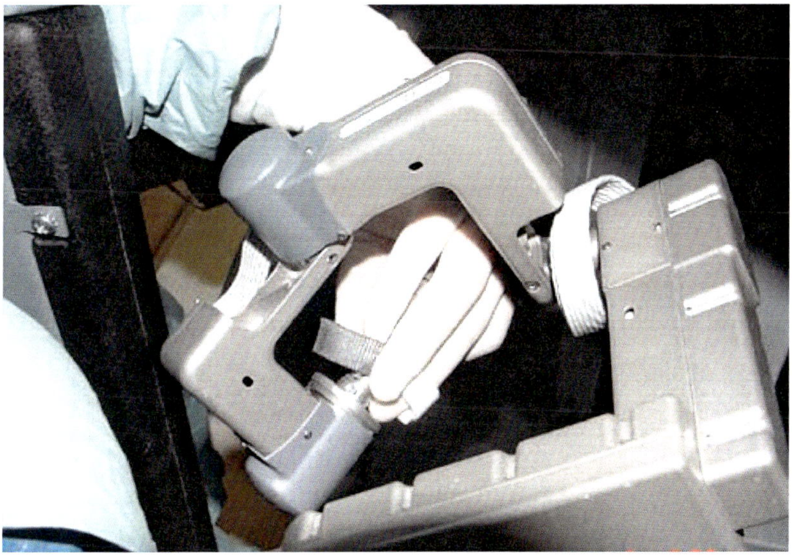

The surgeon inserts his hands into a "master" that translates motions of his hands into motions of the robotic arms and hand-like instruments. The surgeon acts as the "master" and the robot as the "slave" in this telerobotic "master-slave" system. Da Vinci only duplicates the motions of the surgeon. Da Vinci does not initiate any actions on its own volition.

©2010 Intuitive Surgical, Inc.

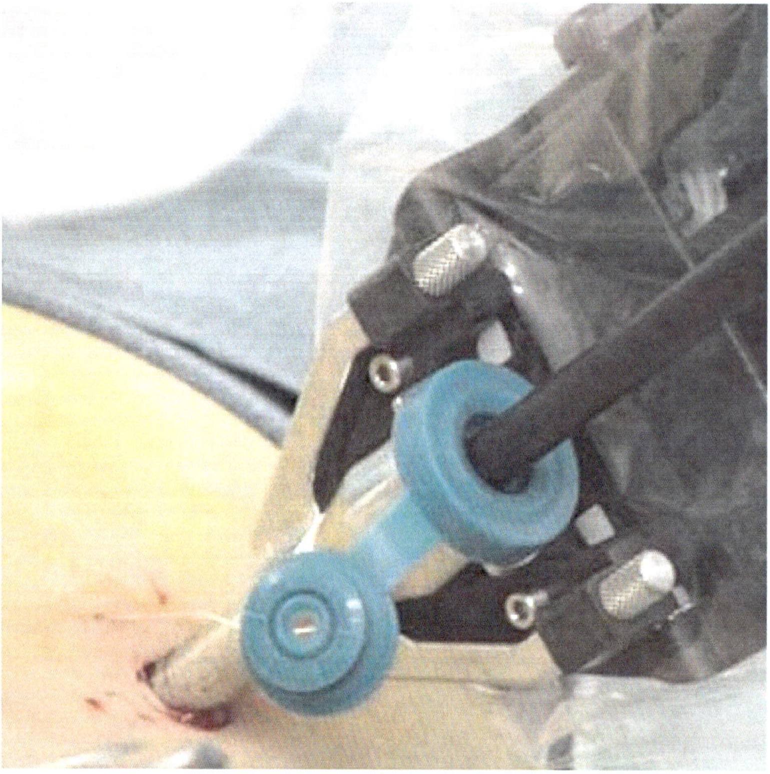

A robotic arm attached to the trocar port, with an instrument in place.

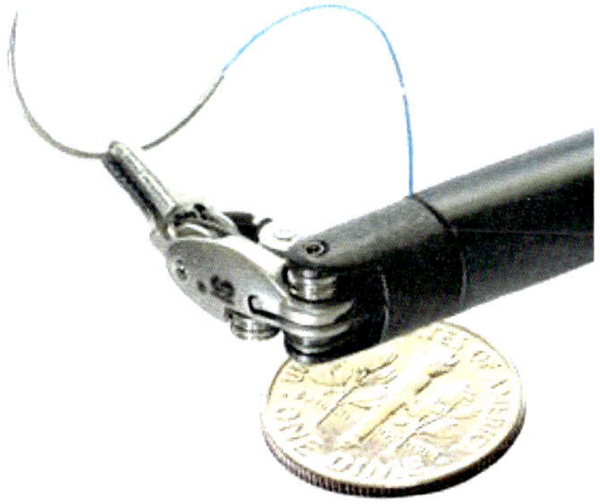

Suturing is all done by dime-sized instruments under the command and use of the joystick in the hands of the skilled surgeon at the console.

Part Four

Recovery from Robotic Surgery

10

What to Expect after Robotic Surgery

BECAUSE DA VINCI ROBOTIC SURGERY is performed through very small incisions; it is associated with minimal surgical pain. Most patients recover without narcotic medication, and this reduces side effects such as dizziness, lethargy, and constipation. The reduction of pain also permits most patients to stand on their feet and walk within hours following surgery and to leave the hospital on the first postoperative day.

Patients generally wake up feeling tired and with a certain amount of pain - this will depend on several factors, including the type of hysterectomy, the reason for it, and the state of health of the patient. Most likely the patient will also be on an IV drip and will have a urinary catheter for a few hours after surgery. The IV drip will usually be discontinued once the patient is eating and drinking normally, usually within a few hours to one to two days.

Patients are usually encouraged to walk soon after surgery; this is to reduce the risk of blood clots in the legs. By the first day after surgery, most patients are walking around. Most women who have had a robotic hysterectomy can safely go home from the hospital within twenty-four hours after surgery.

It is important for the patient not to put anything in her vagina for at least the first six weeks. This includes douching, tampons or having sex. Sometimes, a surgeon may prescribe a vaginal estrogen preparation to help with healing. This preparation may be placed in the vagina if directed by the surgeon.

In the majority of cases, a follow-up appointment will be arranged for about six weeks after the operation. During this period, patients should remain aware of any symptoms that might suggest a problem related to surgery. These symptoms include: fevers over 101.5 degrees, worsening abdominal pain not helped with narcotic pain medications, inability to urinate, pass gas or have a bowel movement, nausea and vomiting, leg swelling, or leg pain. Patients need to need to speak to the surgeon if they have any of these symptoms in the six weeks following surgery. Vaginal or incisional bleeding requiring frequent pad or dressing changes should also be reported promptly to the surgeon. Be sure to get the surgeon's contact information before you leave the hospital, in case you need to contact them for any reason.

For a period of six to eight weeks the patient's body is recovering, and she should not carry any heavy items or undertake physically demanding tasks.

Side Effects

After surgery there may be painful abdominal gas. This will gradually ease up, and can be eased by walking and drinking hot beverages. If it lingers, tell your doctor; there are medications to treat it.

Patients often experience a brownish-red vaginal discharge. This usually continues for several weeks after the operation. It's normal. Sanitary pads can be used after the surgery. The discharge should not have a foul smell or contain pus. The doctor should be notified if this is the case as it could be due to an infection.

Menopausal symptoms may result from surgery. Women who have had their ovaries removed prior to menopause will likely experience severe menopausal symptoms for several days. These may include hot flashes, confusion, sweating, anxiety, and a desire to cry. Some patients may be given hormone replacement therapy (HRT), tablets, patches, or implants. These will start having an effect within a few days.

Body Weight Increase

Some patients gain weight after a hysterectomy. Surgeons insist that it is not the operation itself that may cause this, but rather because of post-operative lack of physical activity. Patients who eat a well-balanced diet, while at the same time watching their calorie intake, will not put on weight. If patients decide to participate in any type of physical exercise, it is important to tell the medical team.

Other Rare Issues

The risk of problems related to a hysterectomy is among the lowest for major surgery. If problems do occur, they may include the following:

- Blood clots in the lungs or leg veins
- Infection
- Bleeding - possibly during or after surgery
- Bowel blockage
- Urinary tract injury
- Problems with the anesthesia

The surgeon will make every effort to reduce the risk of these occurrences with the use of medications, good surgical technique, intra-operative surveillance, and post-operative vigilance. It is important for a patient to know the symptoms associated with each of these so that if they occur, she can alert her surgeon immediately.

Symptoms of blood clots include leg swelling and shortness of breath with a racing heart. Symptoms of infection include fever, redness and/or yellow/green discharge from around the surgical incisions, and foul-smelling vaginal discharge. Bowel blockage symptoms include severe, worsening nausea and vomiting. (Many women will experience nausea in the first few days after surgery, but this should get better quickly.) Urinary tract injury can be signaled by back pain, inability to urinate, blood in the urine, or a constant need to urinate. Symptoms of anesthesia problems include persistent throat soreness. The surgeon should be contacted promptly if any of the above symptoms occur.

What to Expect

Different patients recuperate from robotic hysterectomy at different rates, but a one-night hospital stay is typical. During the hospital stay, the patient is closely monitored to assess pain and ensure comfort. She may receive medications to limit any pain and prevent infection. Light vaginal bleeding is common following robotic hysterectomy.

Hysterectomy patients will no longer experience menstrual periods. If surgeons remove the ovaries, immediate menopause also takes place. The immediate symptoms of menopause include "hot flashes" and mood swings. These symptoms can be treated successfully with estrogen replacement therapy. Patients should discuss the pros and cons associated with estrogen replacement therapy (ERT) with their doctor. Of course, if the patient has already undergone menopause, she will not experience any change in symptoms after hysterectomy.

While many women recover quickly from robotic hysterectomy, some may need up to six to eight weeks for a full surgical recovery. Getting plenty of rest, limiting physical activity, and avoiding heavy lifting are essential during recovery. The patient can generally expect to return to work two to four weeks following robotic surgery.

As with any surgery, patients should consult with their doctors about safely resuming physical activities.

Diet

Clear liquids such as Jell-O, broth, or juices (no soda or carbonated beverages) are recommended until the patient is regularly passing gas without difficulty, or until there has been a good bowel movement. The patient may then resume a regular diet. Avoiding gas-producing foods, such as beans and broccoli is still recommended until you have fully recovered from your surgery.

Activity Level

- Walking and climbing stairs are good and should be done as often as possible.
- Do not sit or lie in one place for long periods of time, other than at bedtime.
- A donut-shaped pillow may provide comfort while sitting.
- Absolutely no biking, motorcycling, or horseback riding for four weeks.
- No sex or vaginal insertions for six to eight weeks.
- Patients may shower twenty-four hours after surgery. No tub baths, swimming or hot tubs for four weeks after surgery.
- Do not drive while taking narcotic pain medications.

Skin Integrity

- There will be four to five port sites (small incisions that the doctor performs the surgery through) that will have Steri-strips (small pieces of tape), and/or Band-Aids over them. Most surgeons use surgical glue or dissolvable sutures to close the small skin incisions. Surgical staples are almost never used.

- Band-Aids may come off in forty-eight hours. Steri-strips may also come off as early as forty-eight hours post-surgery or they may stay in place until you are seen again by the doctor.
- Once the dressings are off, it is not uncommon to have a very small amount of drainage from the incision sites.
- It is normal to have some bruising of the skin on the abdominal wall. This can develop anywhere from one to five days past the surgery. Although it can look scary, it is rarely anything to worry about and resolves in a few weeks.

Clothing:
After surgery, the abdomen may be bloated. It is recommended that recovering patients wear pants with an elastic waist for comfort.

Medications:

- It is possible to resume daily medications as soon as the patient is discharged from the hospital. The only exception to this is Coumadin which is generally resumed after the Foley catheter is removed. The surgeon's instructions should be followed regarding how to resume taking regular medications.
- An antibiotic may be prescribed, to be taken by mouth. If so, the doctor will provide instructions on how to take it.
- An anti-inflammatory pain medication will be prescribed, to be taken by mouth daily. An additional stronger pain medication will be prescribed to use if needed. These prescriptions will be provided on the day of discharge from the hospital.
- A medication to reduce the frequency and severity of bladder spasms may also be prescribed if needed.
- A stool softener should be taken by mouth two times daily. Senakot-S and Colace are good choices. These can be purchased over-the-counter and do not need a prescription. All

narcotic pain medications are constipating and a stool softener will help to prevent this.

Leg/Ankle Swelling

Leg and ankle swelling are usually not abnormal and should not cause alarm. It should resolve in about seven days. Elevating the legs while sitting will help. However, if one leg or ankle is swelling more than the other, this may mean that there is a blood clot. It is very important that the surgeon is notified if this happens during the recovery period.

Avoid Heavy Lifting

The patient may feel great after surgery, but she should not assume that she is in shape for heavy work. The body requires rest and time to allow the surgery to heal. Recovering patients should not lift anything heavier than ten to fifteen pounds for at least six weeks. It is okay for the patient to return to work fairly soon after surgery if the patient's job does not require heavy lifting or fast movements.

Keep in mind that the body is a marvelous instrument that heals and returns to normal when given a small amount of time to recover from surgery. The patient should not expect to rebound and immediately return to her usual self within the first few weeks after surgery. It takes time to heal.

11

Sex after Robotic Surgery

THE EMOTIONAL AND SEXUAL EFFECT OF SURGERY is sometimes troubling. Most women will feel some sadness and a sense of loss after a hysterectomy. Doctors say the emotional impact may be stronger among women of child-bearing age with cancer whose only option was a hysterectomy.

Pre-menopausal women who have a hysterectomy may have a sad feeling that a milestone in life arrived too early - not being able to have children any more. In some cases, this can progress to a feeling of no longer being "womanly," which may progress to clinical depression.

It is important that any mental or emotional symptoms are reported to the doctor if they either persist or grow. Doctors may not only be able to provide treatment, but they may also be able to direct the patient to support groups. Meeting other women who share similar experiences and feelings can be a great help.

Sexual Effects of a Hysterectomy

During a hysterectomy (when the total uterus is removed, including the cervix), the top of the vagina is stitched closed to make a vaginal cuff. This area is full of stitches that require healing. Hysterectomy patients are told "nothing in the vagina" for six to eight weeks and/or until the doctor examines the stitched vaginal cuff during a routine post-op exam and sees it healing properly.

Post-op hysterectomy patients also tend to experience a heightened sense of libido during this time, which makes waiting all the more frustrating. Libido or not, hysterectomy patients should not put ANYTHING into their vagina until released by their personal doctor for sexual intercourse. Sexual intercourse can introduce bacteria into the vagina and cause an infection. Sexual intercourse can also cause torn stitches.

There are reports of women who failed to heed counsel and had to have additional surgery to repair the vaginal cuff, which was torn open by premature sexual intercourse. Some have reported serious infections that put them back in the hospital for antibiotics via IV. Patients have reported bleeding and pain, which required pain medications for days after sex when they did not follow the doctor's orders.

It is important to curtail all vaginal sexual activities until the doctor makes an examination and gives permission to have sexual intercourse. Oral sex can introduce bacteria into the area, so it is not permitted until healing has taken place. Anal sex is also generally not allowed.

Allowing sufficient time to heal is important. Even at the six-week mark, many patients are still told they must wait for sexual activities. Vaginal cuffs that are not healing properly are treated (usually with silver nitrate) and patients are told to wait for an additional two to four weeks.

Change in Sexual Gratification

Some patients may notice a difference in how they respond to sex after the operation. Uterine contractions which were present during orgasm will no longer be there, giving the orgasm a different sensation.

Some patients discover that sex after the surgery is more enjoyable. This could be due to many factors, among which is surely the absence of concern about pregnancy.

Researchers from University of Auckland in New Zealand found that women who undergo a total hysterectomy, in which both the uterus and the cervix are removed, are no more likely to experience sexual difficulties or urinary or bowel problems after surgery than women who have only their uterus removed.

Hormone Therapy

For women who were having regular periods prior to hysterectomy, removal of uterus and ovaries can cause a sudden onset of hot flashes, and emotional swings associated with menopause. These symptoms may be reduced with hormone replacement therapy. If a woman is premenopausal at the time of hysterectomy, she should ask her surgeon about the possibility of hormone replacement therapy.

Instructions for Pleasurable Sex after a Hysterectomy

After a hysterectomy, sex can be as pleasurable as it was before. Women should follow their surgeon's instructions on when to resume having intercourse. This is usually within six to eight weeks after the procedure. Other types of sexual activity may be possible sooner. Patients who experience vaginal dryness during sex can use a lubricant. Be aware that a hysterectomy prevents pregnancy but does not protect against sexually transmitted diseases. A woman should discuss her concerns with her partner and her doctor.

Being Aware of Emotions

After a hysterectomy, a patient may feel relieved to be free of symptoms. She may also feel sad about the changes in her body. If the ovaries were removed, there may be some natural mood swings as the hormones adjust. Mention these mood changes to the doctor if there is concern.

Ongoing Healthcare

Regular physical exams help to ensure general health and well-being.

- You will continue to need routine breast exams and pelvic exams. This may also include Pap smear tests.
- If you're taking HT (Hormone Therapy), you will need follow-up visits with your doctor to fine-tune your dosage.

Part Five

Patient Satisfaction and Questions

12
Letter Excerpts from Actual Patients

THE FOLLOWING ARE VERIFIABLE letter responses to women who have had the da Vinci Robotic Surgery performed:

"On June 24, I went in for my surgery with the da Vinci Surgical System; on July 5, I was holding my daughter and walking down the aisle at my sister-in-law's wedding." Shannon

"None of my friends can believe that I had no pain after my surgery and that I was up and about the next day. I didn't drive for a few days after the surgery, but other than that everything was good." Stacy

"I have spoken to friends who had the traditional hysterectomy, and my experience was so much easier and less painful. I highly recommend it." Lauren

"After a life of regular, painless periods, I was well into what I considered menopause or at least peri-menopause. I had not had a period in about 6 months when bleeding began. Because I had an annual exam already scheduled, I saw my regular ob-gyn within 3-4 weeks of the first sign of bleeding. After an ultrasound, a biopsy, and a D&C,

the word came that I had endometrial cancer (hopefully, low-grade, slow growing).

As soon as hysterectomy was mentioned, my registered nurse friend found the da Vinci web site, and I never looked back. I found my doctor through this site and cannot express what a comfort and wealth of knowledge he was. After an excruciating wait for surgery, I went to Baptist Hospital in Jacksonville on 04/16/09, hoping that da Vinci would work but knowing there was that possibility that a traditional hysterectomy might be required. Well, I woke up to discover that the da Vinci was a resounding Success." Robin

"There is no comparison between conventional surgery and the da Vinci Surgery." Mary

13

What You Would Like to Know

THESE ARE SOME OF THE QUESTIONS that most patients ask concerning robotic surgery:

Q. What is Minimally Invasive Surgery (MIS)?

A. MIS is surgery typically performed through small incisions, or operating ports, rather than large incisions. This can potentially result in shorter recovery times, fewer complications, reduced hospitalization costs and reduced trauma to the patient. While MIS has become the standard-of-care for particular surgical procedures, it has not been widely adopted for more complex or delicate procedures. Robotic surgery makes it easier for more surgeons to adopt minimally invasive surgery to perform procedures like hysterectomy.

Q. Why do we need a new way to do minimally invasive surgery?

A. Despite the widespread use of minimally invasive or laparoscopic surgery in today's hospitals, adoption of laparoscopic techniques, for the most part, has been limited to a few routine procedures. This is due mostly to the limited capabilities of traditional laparoscopic technology, including standard video and rigid instruments, which surgeons must rely on to operate through small incisions. In addition, the extended learning period and the need to "think backwards" have hindered widespread adoption of traditional laparoscopic surgery. Robotic surgery permits the surgeon to perform surgery in an ergonomically comfortable environment, while allowing for improved visualization with magnification, and natural hand movements to achieve outstanding results.

Q. What are the benefits of da Vinci Surgery compared with traditional methods of surgery?

A. Some of the major benefits experienced by surgeons using the *da Vinci* Surgical System over traditional approaches have been greater surgical precision, increased range of motion, improved dexterity, enhanced visualization and improved access.

Benefits experienced by patients may include a shorter hospital stay, less pain, less risk of infection, less blood loss, fewer transfusions, less scarring, faster recovery and a quicker return to normal daily activities. None of these benefits can be guaranteed, as surgery is necessarily both patient and procedure-specific.

Q: Where is the da Vinci Surgical System being used now?

A. Currently, the *da Vinci* Surgical System is being used in hundreds of locations worldwide, in major centers in the United States, Austria, Belgium, Canada, Denmark, France, Germany, Italy, India, Japan, the Netherlands, Romania, Saudi Arabia, Singapore, Sweden, Switzerland, United Kingdom, Australia and Turkey.

Q. Has the da Vinci Surgical System been cleared by the FDA?

A. The U.S. Food and Drug Administration (FDA) has cleared the *da Vinci* Surgical System for a wide range of procedures. In particular, the *da Vinci* system is FDA-approved for gynecologic surgery, including hysterectomy.

Q: Is da Vinci Surgery covered by insurance?

A. *da Vinci* Surgery is categorized as robot-assisted minimally invasive surgery, so any insurance that covers minimally invasive surgery generally covers *da Vinci* Surgery. This is true for widely held insurance plans like Medicare. It is important to note that your coverage will depend on your plan and benefits package. For specifics regarding reimbursement for *da Vinci* surgery, or if you have been denied coverage, please call the Reimbursement Hotline at 1-888-868-4647 ext. 3128. From outside the United States, please call 33-1-39-04-26-90.

Q. Will the da Vinci Surgical System make the surgeon unnecessary?

A. No, the *da Vinci* System enables surgeons to be more precise, advancing their technique and enhancing their capability in performing complex minimally invasive surgery. The system replicates the surgeon's movements in real time. It cannot be programmed, nor can it make decisions on its own to move in any way or perform any type of surgical maneuver without the surgeon's input.

Q. Is a surgeon using the da Vinci Surgical System operating in "virtual reality?"

A. No. Although seated at a console a few feet away from the patient, the surgeon views an actual image of the surgical field while operating in real-time, through tiny incisions, using miniaturized, wristed instruments. At no time does the surgeon see a virtual image or program or command the system to perform any maneuver on its own, outside of the surgeon's direct, real-time control.

Q. Is this telesurgery? Can you operate over long distances?
A. The *da Vinci* Surgical System can theoretically be used to operate over long distances. This capability, however, is not the primary focus, and is not available with the current *da Vinci* Surgical System.

Q. While using the da Vinci Surgical System, can the surgeon feel anything inside the patient's abdomen?
A. Technically, no. However, because of the advanced visualization, many advanced *da Vinci* surgeons report the sense of "feeling the tissues" while operating. This is probably due to visual cues provided by the advanced stereoscopic vision system.

Q: What procedures have been performed using the da Vinci Surgical System? What additional procedures are possible?
A. The *da Vinci* System is a robotic surgical platform designed to enable complex procedures of all types to be performed through one to two centimeter incisions, or operating "ports." To date, tens of thousands of procedures including general, urologic, gynecologic, thoracoscopic, and thoracoscopically-assisted cardiotomy procedures have been performed using the *da Vinci* Surgical System.

Q. Why is it called the da Vinci Surgical System?
A. The product is called "*da Vinci*" in part because Leonardo da Vinci invented the first robot. He also used unparalleled anatomical accuracy and three-dimensional details to bring his masterpieces to life. The *da Vinci* Surgical System similarly provides physicians with such enhanced detail and precision that the System can simulate an open surgical environment while allowing operation through tiny incisions.

Part Six

Alternatives to Hysterectomy

14

Alternative Treatment Options

Nonsurgical treatment options exist for many of the conditions that are treatable with hysterectomy. Most doctors recommend conservative (i.e., non-surgical) therapy as a first line for many of the non-cancerous conditions related to the uterus. When conservative measures fail, surgical therapies can be considered.

Alternatives to hysterectomy

For alternatives to hysterectomy for uterine fibroids including myomectomy, uterine fibroid embolization, Exablate and other treatments, the reader is referred to http://www.fibroid.com

If a woman has fibroids but does not have any symptoms, she may not need treatment. If symptoms are present (e.g., heavy bleeding, pain, pressure), the following should be considered:

- Whether pregnancy may be desired in the future.
- The size of the fibroids.
- The location of the fibroids.
- The patient's age and how close to menopause she is.

There are multiple non-surgical options for management of uterine fibroids, including:

- Medical therapy
- MR Guided Ultrasound Ablation
- GnRH agonists or "Lupron"
- Uterine Fibroid Ablation (UFE)
- Myomectomy

If symptoms include abnormal uterine bleeding, treatment options can include:

- Dilation and Curettage (D & C)
- Lysteda
- Mirena Intrauterine System
- Endometrial ablation
- Progesterone therapy
- Natural therapies

Treatment options for prolapse include:

- Pessaries

Treatment options for endometriosis and adenomyosis include:

- Oral contraceptive therapy
- Hormone therapy
- Non Steroidal anti-inflammatory medication (e.g., Ibuprofen, Naproxen)

Treatment options for pelvic inflammatory disease include:

- Oral and/or intravenous antibiotic therapy

Treatment option(s) for cancer include:

- Radiation - cervical and endometrial cancer only
- Chemotherapy, usually associated with surgical therapy.

Medical Therapy

If mild fibroid symptoms are present, the doctor may suggest taking medication. Over-the-counter drugs such as ibuprofen or acetaminophen can be used for mild pain. An iron supplement can be taken to prevent or correct anemia if there is heavy menstrual bleeding.

Several drugs commonly used for birth control can be prescribed to help control symptoms of fibroids. Low-dose birth control pills do not make fibroids grow and can help control heavy bleeding. The same is true of progesterone-like injections (e.g., Depo-Provera®). An IUD (intrauterine device) called Mirena® contains a small amount of progesterone-like medication, which can be used to control heavy bleeding as well as for birth control.

Other drugs used to treat fibroids are "gonadotropin releasing hormone agonists" (GnRHa). The one most commonly used is Lupron®. These drugs, given by injection, nasal spray, or implanted, can shrink fibroids. Sometimes they are used before surgery to make fibroids easier to remove. Side effects of GnRHas can include hot flashes, depression, not being able to sleep, decreased sex drive, and joint pain. Most women tolerate GnRHas quite well. Most women do not get a period when taking GnRHas. This can be a big relief to women who have heavy bleeding.

It also allows women with anemia to recover to a normal blood count. GnRHas can cause bone thinning, so their use is generally limited to six months or less. These drugs also are very expensive, and some insurance companies will cover only some or none of the cost. GnRHas offers temporary relief from the symptoms of fibroids; once you stop taking the drugs, the fibroids often grow back quickly.

A new drug, LYSTEDA™, was recently approved by the FDA for the treatment of Heavy Menstrual Bleeding (HMB). LYSTEDA is a non-hormonal medication that is taken only during menstruation, as opposed to every day. LYSTEDA cannot be used as birth control, and because it does not contain hormones, it doesn't have hormonal side effects. LYSTEDA was also shown to help make a meaningful difference as early as the first menstrual cycle and for all cycles studied.

When nonsurgical therapies fail to produce satisfactory results, and a woman does not desire future fertility, hysterectomy may be a suitable next step for treating the conditions discussed above. Robotic surgery offers a safe, comprehensive, minimally invasive approach to hysterectomy, allowing the woman to return to normal activities quickly, with minimal pain and discomfort.

Part Seven

Glossary and Safety Information,

Glossary of Terms

amenorrhea - absence or cessation of menstrual periods.

amenorrhea, primary - from the beginning and lifelong; menstruation never begins at puberty.

amenorrhea, secondary - due to some physical cause and usually of later onset; a condition in which menstrual periods which were at one time normal and regular become increasing abnormal and irregular or absent.

anovulation - failure of the ovaries to produce or release mature eggs.

benign - cell growth that is not cancerous, does not invade nearby tissue, or spread to other parts of the body.

biological therapy (Also called immunotherapy, biotherapy, or

biological response modifier therapy.) - uses the body's immune system, either directly or indirectly, to fight cancer or to lessen side effects that may be caused by some cancer treatments.

biopsy - removal of sample of tissue via a hollow needle or scalpel.

cancer - abnormal cells that divide without control, which can invade nearby tissues or spread through the bloodstream and lymphatic system to other parts of the body.

carcinogen - a substance that is known to cause cancer.

cervicitis - an irritation of the cervix by a number of different organisms. Cervicitis is generally classified as either acute or chronic.

cervix - the lower, narrow part of the uterus (womb) located between the bladder and the rectum. It forms a canal that opens into the vagina, which leads to the outside of the body.

chemotherapy - treatment to destroy cancer cells with drugs.

chlamydial infection - very common sexually transmitted disease or urinary tract infection caused by a bacteria-like organism in the urethra and reproductive system.

climacteric (Also called perimenopause.) - the transition period of time before menopause, marked by a decreased production of estrogen and progesterone, irregular menstrual periods, and transitory psychological changes.

clinical trials - organized research studies that provide clinical data aimed at finding better ways to prevent, detect, diagnose, or treat diseases.

cold knife cone biopsy - a procedure in which a laser or a surgical scalpel is used to remove a piece of tissue. This procedure requires the use of general anesthesia.

colony-stimulating factors - substances that stimulate the production of blood cells.

colposcopy (Also called colposcopic biopsy.) - a procedure which uses an instrument with magnifying lenses, called a colposcope, to examine the cervix for abnormalities. If abnormal tissue is found, a biopsy is usually performed.

computed tomography (Also called CT or CAT scan.) - a non-invasive procedure that takes cross-sectional images of the brain or other internal organs; to detect any abnormalities that may not show up on an ordinary x-ray. The CT scan may indicate enlarged lymph nodes - a possible sign of a spreading cancer or of an infection.

cone biopsy (Also called conization.) - a biopsy in which a larger cone-shaped piece of tissue is removed from the cervix by using the loop electrosurgical excision procedure or the cold knife cone biopsy procedure. The cone biopsy procedure may be used as a treatment for precancerous lesions and early cancers.

cryosurgery - use of liquid nitrogen, or a probe that is very cold, to freeze and kill cancer cells.

culdocentesis - a procedure in which a needle is inserted into the pelvic cavity through the vaginal wall to obtain a sample of pus.

cyst - a fluid-filled or semi-solid sac in or under the skin.

cystitis - inflammation of the urinary bladder and ureters.

dilation and curettage (D & C) - a minor operation in which the cervix is dilated (expanded) so that the cervical canal and uterine lining can be scraped with a curette (spoon-shaped instrument).

dysmenorrhea - pain or discomfort experienced just before or during a menstrual period.

dysmenorrhea, primary - from the beginning and usually lifelong; severe and frequent menstrual cramping caused by uterine contractions.

dysmenorrhea, secondary - due to some physical cause and usually of later onset; painful menstrual periods caused by another medical condition present in the body (i.e., pelvic inflammatory disease, endometriosis).

dyspareunia - pain in the vagina or pelvis experienced during sexual intercourse.

ectopic pregnancy (Also called tubal pregnancy.) - pregnancy that develops outside the uterus, usually in one of the fallopian tubes.

endocervical curettage (ECC) - a procedure which uses a narrow instrument called a curette to scrape the lining of the endocervical canal. This type of biopsy is usually completed along with the colposcopic biopsy.

endometrial ablation - a procedure to destroy the lining of the uterus (endometrium).

endometrial biopsy - a procedure in which a sample of tissue is obtained through a tube which is inserted into the uterus.

endometrial hyperplasia - abnormal thickening of the endometrium caused by excessive cell growth.

endometrial implants - fragments of endometrium that relocate outside of the uterus, such as in the muscular wall of the uterus, ovaries, fallopian tubes, vagina, or intestine.

endometrial resection - a procedure to remove the lining of the uterus (endometrium).

endometriosis - condition in which tissue resembling that of the endometrium grows outside the uterus, on or near the ovaries or fallopian tubes, or in other areas of the pelvic cavity.

endometrium - mucous membrane lining of the inner surface of the uterus that grows during each menstrual cycle and is shed in menstrual blood.

endoscopy - use of a very flexible tube with a lens or camera (and a light on the end), which is connected to a computer screen, allowing the physician to see inside the hollow organs, such as the uterus. Biopsy samples can be taken through the tube.

estrogen - a group of hormones secreted by the ovaries which affect many aspects of the female body, including a woman's menstrual cycle and normal sexual and reproductive development.

Estrogen therapy (ERT) - use of the female hormone estrogen to replace that which the body no longer produces naturally after medical or surgical menopause.

excisional - cutting away cancerous tissue with a scalpel or other instruments to completely remove it and possibly some surrounding tissue. There are many types of excisional surgeries, each named for the particular area of the body in which they are performed, or the particular purpose for which they are performed.

expectant management (expectant therapy) - "watchful waiting" or close monitoring of a disease by a physician instead of immediate treatment.

extragenital - outside of, away from, unrelated to the genital organs.

fallopian tubes - two thin tubes that extend from each side of the uterus, toward the ovaries, as a passageway for eggs and sperm.

fecal occult blood test - test to check for hidden blood in stool.

fertile - able to become pregnant.

fibroids - noncancerous growths in, on, or within the walls of the uterus.

fibroid embolization - a new minimally-invasive (without a large abdominal incision) technique which involves identifying which arteries are supplying blood to the fibroids and then blocking off these arteries, which cuts off the fibroids blood supply and causes them to shrink. Physicians are still evaluating the long-term implications of this procedure on fertility and regrowth of the fibroid.

follicle-stimulating hormone (FSH) - hormone secreted by the pituitary gland in the brain that stimulates the growth and maturation of eggs in females and sperm in males, and sex hormone production in both males and females.

genital herpes - a sexually transmitted disease caused by the herpes simplex virus.

genital warts - a sexually transmitted disease caused by the human papillomavirus (HPV).

genitals - external sex organs.

grading - a process for classifying cancer cells to determine the growth rate of the tumor. The cancer cells are measured by how closely they look like normal cells.

hirsutism - excess growth of body and facial hair, including the chest, stomach, and back

hormone therapy (HRT) - use of the female hormones estrogen and progestin (a synthetic form of progesterone) to replace those hormones the body no longer produces after menopause.

hormone therapy - treatment of cancer by removing, blocking, or adding hormones.

hormones - chemical substances created by the body that control numerous body functions.

human papillomaviruses (HPVs) - a group of viruses that can cause warts. Some HPVs are sexually transmitted and cause wart-like growths on the genitals. HPV is associated with some types of cancer.

hyperplasia - an abnormal increase in the number of cells in a tissue or an organ (i.e., cervix or the lining of the uterus).

hysterectomy - surgery to remove the uterus.

hysterosalpingography - x-ray examination of the uterus and fallopian tubes that uses dye and is often performed to rule out tubal obstruction.

hysteroscopy - visual examination of the canal of the cervix and the interior of the uterus using a viewing instrument (hysteroscope) inserted through the vagina.

imaging - tests or evaluation procedures that produce pictures of areas inside the body.

immune system - group of organs, antibodies, and cells that defends the body against infection or disease.

immunotherapy (Also called biological therapy.) - treatment that uses the body's natural defenses to fight cancer.

infertility - unable to produce children.

interferon - a biological response modifier that stimulates the growth of certain disease-fighting blood cells in the immune system.

interleukin-2 - a biological response modifier that stimulates the growth of certain blood cells in the immune system that can fight cancer.

invasive cancer - cancer that begins in one area and then spreads deeper into the tissues of that area.

labia - the folds of skin at the opening of the vagina (and other organs).

laparoscopic lymph node sampling - lymph nodes are removed through a viewing tube called a laparoscope, which is inserted through a small incision in the abdomen.

laparoscopy - use of a viewing tube with a lens or camera (and a light on the end), which is inserted through a small incision in the abdomen to examine the contents of the abdomen and remove tissue samples.

laparotomy - a surgical procedure that involves an incision from the upper to lower abdomen; often used when making a diagnosis by less invasive tests is difficult.

loop electrosurgical excision procedure (LEEP) - a procedure which uses an electric wire loop to obtain a piece of tissue.

luteinizing hormone (LH) - hormone secreted by the pituitary gland in the brain that stimulates the growth and maturation of eggs in females and sperm in males.

lymph nodes (Also called lymph glands.) - small organs located in the channels of the lymphatic system which store special cells to trap bacteria or cancer cells traveling through the body in lymph. Clusters of lymph nodes are found in the underarms, groin, neck, chest, and abdomen.

lymphatic system - tissues and organs, including bone marrow, spleen, thymus, and lymph nodes, that produce, store, and carry white blood cells to fight infection and disease.

magnetic resonance imaging (MRI) - a non-invasive procedure that produces a two-dimensional view of an internal organ or structure, especially the brain and spinal cord. The MRI may show abnormal nodules in bones or lymph nodes - a sign that cancer may be spreading.

malignant - cancerous cells are present.

mammogram - x-ray of the breast tissue.

menarche - a young woman's first menstrual period.

menopause - end of menstruation; commonly used to refer to the period ending the female reproductive phase of life.

menorrhagia - the most common type of abnormal uterine bleeding (also called dysfunctional uterine bleeding) characterized by heavy and prolonged menstrual bleeding. In some cases, bleeding may be so severe and relentless that daily activities become interrupted.

menses - menstrual flow.

menstruation - a cyclical process of the endometrium shedding its lining, along with discharge from the cervix and vagina, from the vaginal opening. This process results from the mature egg cell (ovum) not being fertilized by a sperm cell as it travels from one of the ovaries down a fallopian tube to the uterus, in the process called ovulation.

metastasis - spread of cancer from one part of the body to another.

metrorrhagia - any irregular, acyclical nonmenstrual bleeding from the uterus; bleeding between menstrual periods.

monoclonal antibodies - substances that can locate and bind to cancer cells wherever they are in the body.

obstetrician/gynecologist (OB/GYN) - physicians who specialize in general women's medical care, diagnosis and treatment of disorders of the female reproductive system, and care of pregnant women.

oligomenorrhea - infrequent or light menstrual cycles.

oncologist - physician who specializes in treating cancer.

oophorectomy - surgery to remove one or both ovaries.

ovaries - two female reproductive organs located in the pelvis.

ovulation - release of a mature egg from an ovary.

ovum - a mature egg cell released during ovulation from an ovary.

Pap test (Also called Pap smear.) - Test that involves microscopic examination of cells collected from the cervix, used to detect changes that may be cancer or may lead to cancer, and to show noncancerous conditions, such as infection or inflammation.

pathologist - physician who identifies diseases by studying cells and tissues under a microscope.

pelvic examination - an internal examination of the uterus, vagina, ovaries, fallopian tubes, bladder, and rectum.

pelvic inflammatory disease (PID) - inflammation of the pelvic organs caused by a type of bacteria.

pelvic lymph node dissection - removal of some lymph nodes from the pelvis.

pelvis - a basin-shaped structure that supports the spinal column and contains the sacrum, coccyx, and hip bones (ilium, pubis, and ischium).

perimenopause (Also called climacteric.) - the transition period of time before menopause, marked by a decreased production of estrogen and progesterone, irregular menstrual periods, and transitory psychological changes.

perineal - related to the perineum.

perineum - area between the anus and the sex organs.

peripheral stem cell support - procedure to replace blood-forming cells destroyed by cancer treatment. Stem cells in the blood that are similar to cells in the bone marrow are removed from the patient's blood before treatment and given back to the patient after treatment.

placenta - organ that develops in the uterus during pregnancy; links the blood supplies of a pregnant woman to the fetus to provide nutrients and remove waste products.

polymenorrhea - too frequent menstruation.

polyps - a growth that projects from the lining of mucous membrane, such as the intestine.

postmenopausal bleeding - any bleeding that occurs more than 6 months after the last normal menstrual period at menopause.

premenstrual dysphoric disorder (PMDD) - a much more severe form of the collective symptoms known as premenstrual syndrome (PMS), premenstrual dysphoric disorder (PMDD) is considered a severe and chronic medical condition that requires attention and treatment.

premenstrual syndrome (PMS) - a group of physical and emotional symptoms that some women experience during their menstrual cycle. Although the symptoms usually cease with onset of the menstrual period, in some women, symptoms may last through and after their menstrual periods.

progesterone - female hormone.

progestin - synthetic form of the female sex hormone progesterone.

radiation therapy (Also called radiotherapy.) - treatment with high-energy rays (such as x-rays or gamma rays) to kill cancer cells; may be by external radiation or by internal radiation from radioactive materials placed directly in or near the tumor.

radionuclide scan - an imaging scan in which a small amount of radioactive substance is injected into the vein. A machine measures levels of radioactivity in certain organs, thereby detecting any abnormal areas or tumors.

rectum - lower end of the large intestine, leading to the anus.

recur - to occur again; reappearance of cancer cells at the same site or in another location.

risk factor - activity or factor that may increase the chance of developing a disease.

salpingectomy - surgical removal of one or both fallopian tubes.

salpingo-oophorectomy - surgery to remove the fallopian tubes and ovaries.

Schiller test - a diagnostic test in which the cervix is coated with an iodine solution to detect the presence of abnormal cells.

sexually transmitted disease (STD) - infection spread through sexual intercourse and other intimate sexual contact.

screening - checking for disease when there are no symptoms.

stage - the extent of a cancer, whether the disease has spread from the original site to other parts of the body.

surgery - operation to remove or repair a part of the body, or to find out if disease is present.

systemic treatment - treatment using substances that travel through the bloodstream and reach cancer cells all over the body.

tamoxifen - an anticancer drug used in hormone therapy to block the effects of estrogen.

tissue - group or layer of cells that together perform specific functions.

total hysterectomy - the removal of the uterus, including the cervix; the fallopian tubes and the ovaries remain.

total hysterectomy with bilateral salpingo-oophorectomy - the entire uterus, fallopian tubes, and the ovaries are surgically removed.

transvaginal ultrasound (Also called ultrasonography.) - an ultrasound test using a small instrument, called a transducer, that is placed in the vagina.

trichomoniasis - very common type of vaginitis caused by a single-celled organism usually transmitted during sexual contact.

tumor - abnormal mass of tissue that results from excessive cell division; may be benign (not cancerous) or malignant (cancerous).

ultrasound - an imaging technique that uses sound waves to produce an image on a monitor of the abdominal organs, such as the uterus, liver, and kidneys.

urethra - narrow channel through which urine passes from the bladder out of the body.

urethritis - infection limited to the urethra.

uterus - also called the womb, the uterus is a hollow, pear-shaped organ located in a woman's lower abdomen, between the bladder and the rectum.

vagina (Also called the birth canal.) - the passageway through which fluid passes out of the body during menstrual periods. The vagina connects the cervix (the opening of the womb, or uterus) and the vulva (the external genitalia).

vaginal atrophy - often a symptom of menopause; the drying and thinning of the tissues of the vagina and urethra. This can lead to dyspareunia (pain during sexual intercourse) as well as vaginitis, cystitis, and urinary tract infections.

vaginal hysterectomy - the uterus is removed through the vaginal opening.

vaginitis - inflammation, redness, or swelling of the vaginal tissues; usually resulting from a bacterial infection.

vaginitis, atrophic - a form of noninfectious vaginitis which usually results from a decrease in hormones because of menopause, surgical removal of the ovaries, radiation therapy, or even after childbirth - particularly in breastfeeding women. Lack of estrogen dries and thins the vaginal tissue, and may also cause spotting.

vaginitis, bacterial - very common vaginal infection characterized by symptoms such as increased vaginal discharge or itching, burning, or redness in the genital area.

vaginitis, noninfectious - a type of vaginitis that usually refers to vaginal irritation without an infection being present. Most often, the infection is caused by an allergic reaction to, or irritation from, vaginal sprays, douches, or spermicidal products. It may also be caused by sensitivity to perfumed soaps, detergents, or fabric softeners.

vaginitis, viral - very common vaginal infection, often sexually transmitted, that is caused by one of many different types of viruses (i.e., herpes simplex virus, human papillomavirus).

vulva - external, visible part of the female genital area.

vulvitis - an inflammation of the vulva, the soft folds of skin outside the vagina. This is not a condition but rather a symptom that results from a host of diseases, infections, injuries, allergies, and other irritants.

white blood cells - cells that help the body fight infection and disease.

x-ray - electromagnetic energy used to produce images of bones and internal organs onto film.

Courtesy Robert Wood Johnson University Hospital

Important Safety Information

Indications for Use

The U.S. Food and Drug Administration (FDA) has cleared the *da Vinci®* Surgical System for use in urological surgical procedures, general laparoscopic surgical procedures, gynecologic laparoscopic surgical procedures, transoral otolaryngology surgical procedures restricted to benign and malignant tumors classified as T1 and T2, general thoracoscopic surgical procedures, and thoracoscopically assisted cardiotomy procedures. The system can also be employed with adjunctive mediastinotomy to perform coronary anastomosis during cardiac revascularization. The system is indicated for adult and pediatric use (except for transoral otolaryngology surgical procedures). It is intended for use by trained physicians in an operating room environment in accordance with representative, specific procedures set forth in the Professional Instructions for Use.

Contraindications for Use

Any and all factors that would make the use of conventional minimally invasive instruments and surgical technique unadvisable also apply to the use of the *da Vinci* Surgical System. General contraindications to minimally invasive surgery may include bleeding disorders, history of prior surgery, pregnancy and significant cardio-pulmonary conditions.

Alternative Treatment Options

Although the *da Vinci* Surgical System is considered safe and effective, it may not be appropriate for every individual, as an individual's circumstances may preclude using minimally invasive techniques or suggest other treatment options. Always ask your doctor about all treatment options that may be appropriate for your medical condition, as well as their risks and benefits. If you have questions about the *da Vinci* Surgical System or a *da Vinci* procedure, consult with a qualified physician familiar with the *da Vinci* Surgical System. A list of physicians experienced with the *da Vinci* Surgical System can be found in the Surgeon Locator section.

Conversion to Non-Minimally Invasive Technique

Environmental or equipment failures may cause the *da Vinci* Surgical System to be unavailable, and may require your doctor to convert to alternative surgical techniques. Ask your doctor about the potential risk of such conversions.

Surgeon Training

The *da Vinci* Surgical System should be used only by surgeons who have developed adequate robotic skills to perform the tasks associated with each procedure and who have received specific training in the use of the *da Vinci* Surgical System. Make sure that your surgeon is well trained in performing hysterectomies, and has special training in the use of the Da Vinci surgical system. Your surgeon should also be skilled at alternative methods of hysterectomy, in case the robotic procedure needs to be converted to an open or laparoscopic approach for any reason. You are encouraged investigate your surgeon's training and experience by searching the American Medical Association's (AMA) "Directory of Physicians in the U.S." and the American Board of Medical Specialties (ABMS) "Official Directory of Board Certified Medical Specialists." For Gynecologists, the certifying board is the American Board of Obstetrics and Gynecology (ABOG), found on the internet at www.abog.org.

Medical Advice Disclaimer

This book is not intended to provide medical advice . If you feel like you have any of the conditions discussed in this book, please contact a qualified physician, who will be able to evaluate you, and offer appropriate treatment advice.

About the Authors

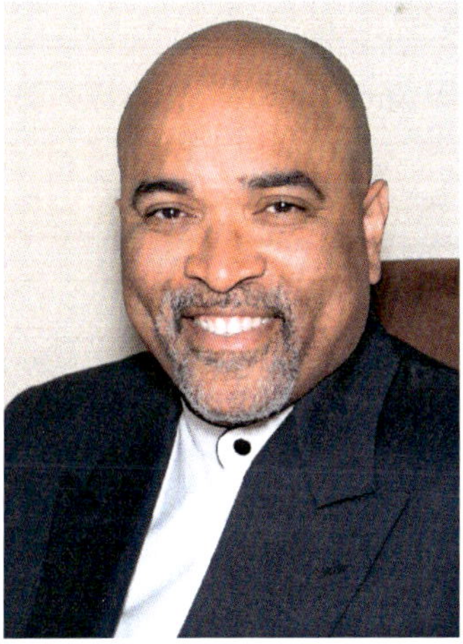

Dr. Lennox Hoyte, MD

Dr. Hoyte is a board certified OB/Gyn physician, and a fellowship trained urogynecologist and pelvic reconstructive surgeon. He is director of the division of urogynecology and pelvic reconstructive surgery at University of South Florida College Of Medicine, and director of urogynecology at Tampa General Hospital. Dr. Hoyte treats women with pelvic organ prolapse, urinary and fecal incontienence, and bladder control problems.

He received his Masters degree in Electrical engineering and Computer science from MIT, and his MD degree from Stanford

Medical School. He received Residency training on OB/Gyn from Brigham and Womens and Massachussetts General Hospitals in Boston, and completed formal fellowship training in Female Pelvic Medicine and Reconstructive Surgery at Loyola University Medical Center in Chicago. He is a Diplomate of the American Board of Obstetrics and Gynecology and a Fellow of the American College of Obstetricians and Gynecologists (ACOG). He is also an elected member of the Society of Gynecologic Surgeons.

Dr. Hoyte was an early user of the Da Vinci Robotic surgical system for gynecologic procedures and has performed over 200 robotic gynecologic surgical procedures. He is the medical director of the USF HEALTH ***Da Vinci*** ® Center for Computer assisted surgery in Tampa, and has trained many surgeons in the use of the Da Vinci surgical system.

He is director of the fellowship training program in urogynecology at USF. He sees patients at the USF physicians group practice in Tampa, and can be reached for appointments at 813-259-8500. He can be reached by email at: urogynmd@mac.com

USF OB/Gyn group
2A Tampa General Circle
Tampa, FL, 33606
Phone Number: (813) 259-8500

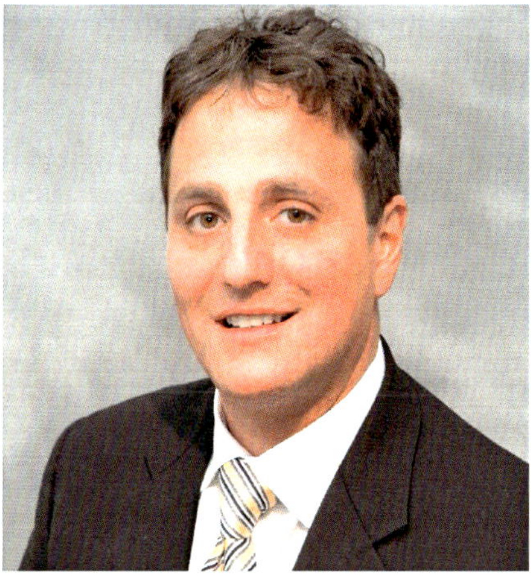

Abraham R. Shashoua, M.D.

Dr. Shashoua is Director of Minimally Invasive and Robotic Gynecologic Surgery at Advocate Illinois Masonic Medical Center. He is board certified in Obstetrics and Gynecology and is a Clinical Assistant Professor in Obstetrics and Gynecology at the University of Illinois. He specializes in urogynecology, minimally invasive procedures and advanced laparoscopy for the management of chronic pelvic pain, pelvic organ prolapse, uterine fibroids, endometriosis, and heavy menstrual bleeding. He is a teaching proctor for the Da Vinci surgical system.

A Chicago native, Dr. Shashoua attended the University of Miami in Florida. He completed medical school at the University of Miami then returned to Chicago to complete a residence in Obstetrics and Gynecology at the University of Chicago. He started in private practice in Chicago and served as Chairman of the Department of Obstetrics and Gynecology at Weiss Memorial Hospital in 2002-2007.

Dr. Shashoua was one of the first in the country to utilize the da Vinci robot for gynecology. He was the first in Chicago to perform a robotic hysterectomy, robotic myomectomy and robotic sacrocolpopexy. Since 2005, he has performed and taught over 500 robotic procedures. He teaches and lectures nationally and internationally on minimally invasive surgery and robotic surgery.

Abraham R. Shashoua, M. D.
3000 North Halsted Street, Suite 405
Chicago, IL 60657
Phone Number: (773) 564-6025